Technology in the Modern Corporation

A Strategic Perspective

Pergamon Titles of Related Interest

Special Issues of Technology in Society

BIOTECHNOLOGY IN SOCIETY, edited by **Joseph G. Perpich**

SCIENCE ADVICE TO THE PRESIDENT, edited by **William T. Golden**

TAXATION, TECHNOLOGY AND THE U.S. ECONOMY, edited by **Ralph Landau** and **N. Bruce Hannay**

TECHNOLOGY AND PHILOSOPHY, edited by **Carl Mitcham**

TECHNOLOGY IN THE MODERN CORPORATION: A STRATEGIC PERSPECTIVE, edited by **Mel Horwitch**

UNIVERSITY-INDUSTRY RESEARCH INTERACTIONS, edited by **Herbert I. Fusfeld** and **Carmela S. Haklisch**

Other Books of Interest

Bernhard et al., SCIENCE, TECHNOLOGY AND SOCIETY IN THE TIME OF ALFRED NOBEL

Bushnell, TRAINING FOR NEW TECHNOLOGY

Dhillon, HUMAN RELIABILITY

Fleissner, SYSTEMS APPROACH TO APPROPRIATE TECHNOLOGY TRANSFER

Heden & King, SOCIAL INNOVATIONS FOR DEVELOPMENT

Hussey, THE TRUTH ABOUT CORPORATE PLANNING

McNulty, INTERNATIONAL DIRECTORY OF EXECUTIVE EDUCATION

Schmeikal et al., IMPACT OF TECHNOLOGY ON SOCIETY

UNESCO, SCIENTIFIC FORECASTING AND HUMAN NEEDS

Related Journals

(Sample copies available on request)

ENERGY CONVERSION AND MANAGEMENT

HUMAN RELIABILITY

INTERNATIONAL JOURNAL OF APPLIED ENGINEERING EDUCATION

JOURNAL OF THE OPERATIONAL RESEARCH SOCIETY

LONG RANGE PLANNING

MATERIALS AND SOCIETY

NUCLEAR AND CHEMICAL WASTE MANAGEMENT

TECHNOLOGY IN SOCIETY

Technology in the Modern Corporation

A Strategic Perspective

Edited by
Mel Horwitch

Alfred P. Sloan School of Management
Massachusetts Institute of Technology

PERGAMON PRESS

New York   Oxford   Beijing   Frankfurt   São Paulo   Sydney   Tokyo   Toronto

Pergamon Press Offices:

U.S.A.	Pergamon Press, Maxwell House, Fairview Park, Elmsford, New York 10523, U.S.A.
U.K.	Pergamon Press, Headington Hill Hall, Oxford OX3 0BW, England
PEOPLE'S REPUBLIC OF CHINA	Pergamon Press, Qianmen Hotel, Beijing, People's Republic of China
FEDERAL REPUBLIC OF GERMANY	Pergamon Press, Hammerweg 6, D-6242 Kronberg-Taunus, Federal Republic of Germany
BRAZIL	Pergamon Editora, Rua Eça de Queiros, 346, CEP 04011, São Paulo, Brazil
AUSTRALIA	Pergamon Press (Aust.) Pty., P.O. Box 544, Potts Point, NSW 2011, Australia
JAPAN	Pergamon Press, 8th Floor, Matsuoka Central Building, 1-7-1 Nishishinjuku, Shinjuku, Tokyo 160, Japan
CANADA	Pergamon Press Canada, Suite 104, 150 Consumers Road, Willowdale, Ontario M2J 1P9, Canada

Published as a special issue of the journal *Technology in Society,* Volume 7, Number 2/3 and supplied to subscribers as part of their normal subscriptions. Also available to non-subscribers.

First printing 1986

Library of Congress Cataloging in Publication Data

Technology in the modern corporation.

    Includes bibliographical references.
    1. Technology. 2. Technological innovations.
3. Industrial management. I. Horwitch, Mel.
T49.5.T443   1986   658.5'14   86-5082
ISBN 0-08-034239-6

Printed in the United States of America

Contents

Preface

Mel Horwitch

The importance of technology in modern society is readily acknowledged. Its profound influence on such societal-level matters as the shape of the modern economy, continued social well-being, and widespread problems is well documented. Moreover, the process of developing technology at the individual, small-group and specialist levels has also been analyzed in depth.

But one of the most active, yet unstudied, domains of technological decision-making today takes place at the firm level—somewhere between the highly macro perspective of society and the micro orientation of the individual or small group.

This special issue of *Technology In Society* is devoted to examining this increasingly important corporate-wide viewpoint which characterizes much of the current technological deliberations. Specifically, this issue views technology with a corporate strategic orientation. Technology is considered from a total-firm and top-level perspective and is seen as playing an essential role in achieving long-term competitive advantage.

The force of technology within the firm is clearly pervasive. Its impact is not limited to the obviously technology-intensive units of a business, such as the industrial R&D facility, nor is concern about technology simply rising to the very top of the enterprise. Instead, there is also a growing interaction between technology and other strategic activities. Technology is affecting various business or product strategies, for example, in suggesting new forms of business or product synergies. Technology is often a key ingredient in formulating functional strategies, including manufacturing, finance, and human resources. Finally, technology is modifying in significant ways the internal structure, processes, and systems of a firm.

These and other general trends can be discerned from the articles in this Special Issue of *Technology In Society*. At least five inter-related major themes emerge. First, it is indeed true that technology is a key part of modern strategic management. Practically all the articles document this fact. In particular, Yves Doz, Reinhard Angelmar and C.K. Prahalad, John Friar and myself, and William Hamilton all emphasize how technology is woven into the strategic decision-making of the technology-intensive corporation. As Michael L. Tushman, Beverly Virany and Elaine Romanelli indicate, CEO attention is important for successful innovation. Graham R. Mitchell presents some sophisticated approaches for technology strategic planning.

A second theme is the important attention being given to structure in often determining the success of technology strategy. It is clear that the dramatic achievements of the small, high-technology, entrepreneurial firm have provided an intriguing model for organizing—at least, partially—innovative activity in the large corporation. Firms are now experimenting with different and multiple kinds of structures for developing technology with small-scale, loosely run units and various types of intra- and inter-organizational linkages being emphasized. These points are discussed throughout this issue, but especially by Robert A. Burgelman, and James Brian Quinn.

A third theme of great importance is that the move toward a strategic view of technology is a global phenomenon. The elevation of technology to a matter of high strategic importance is taking place in Europe and Japan, as well as in the United States. Indeed, some non-US firms, particularly in Japan, appear to be extremely effective in using their technological resources for continuous strategic success. The non-US and global aspects of technology strategy are examined especially by Kiyoshi Kinami, Pedro Nueno and Jan P. Oosterveld, Bruce Rubinger, and D. Eleanor Westney and Kiyonori Sakakibara.

A fourth theme is the significant role of technology in implementing strategy throughout the corporation. A key aspect of this theme is the importance of technology in timing business decisions, such as new product introduction. Richard N. Foster, for example, stresses the power of technology in creating whole new industries and substantially modifying the life-cycles of industries and products.

A final important theme is the changing role of industrial research and development. As competing approaches for developing technology have emerged, that venerable and important institution, the corporate R&D facility, has changed in order to meet new conditions. Margaret B.W. Graham discusses this evolution.

The rise of technology strategy is clearly an important and enduring development that is both widespread and multifaceted. As the articles in this issue indicate, the current practice of viewing technology from a strategic perspective is a new, growing, and fundamental aspect of technological activity in modern society.

Introduction

Technology In Society has always sought to anticipate and to help structure the discussion of major technological issues facing society. In order to fulfill this objective, we have, on occasion, devoted an entire issue to a subject of major importance. These special issues have been well received by our readers; most have been published in book form, widely-cited, and reprinted several times. These issues were made possible by distinguished men and women, who are thoroughly versed in their fields, acquainted with other leaders and contributors, and willing to "volunteer" for the complex and necessary task as Guest Editors.

With each such issue, our intent was to serve as an informed and ready forum for experienced, farsighted and scholarly analysis and views. This issue, "Technology in the Modern Corporation: A Strategic Perspective," represents the most current thinking on the new role of technology in corporate planning and all that this relationship implies to corporate organization and strategy. The issue is among the first collections of research and integrative articles in print dealing with this theme. Although such specific and related areas as technological innovation, management of industrial R&D, and the role of entrepreneurship have been examined in great depth, there has been in the past ten years an inexorable movement towards viewing technology as part of a larger system of activities within the corporation. This development was part of a trend to reexamine the relationships between R&D, human resources, manufacturing, finance, and marketing, and how to integrate these functions more effectively. New insights now have led to the inevitable conclusion that technology has become a strategic variable and must be treated as such.

One of the pioneers in introducing and developing this concept is Professor Mel Horwitch of the Alfred P. Sloan School of Management at the Massachusetts Institute of Technology. We invited Professor Horwitch to assemble in one issue original articles devoted to technology and strategic management. We believe that this issue will inform and be useful to a wide range of readers—policy makers, managers, researchers, and the informed public.

Mel Horwitch teaches strategic management and technology strategy at the Sloan School. He was educated at Princeton University and the Harvard Business School, and has had extensive administrative and consulting experience in business and government throughout the world.

Professor Horwitch has a broad and deep background in the fields of strategic management and the management of technology, and it is natural that he is now at the forefront in merging these fields. His early research focused on specific kinds of technological undertakings. He has written a pioneering book on the American supersonic transport conflict, *Clipped Wings*, and a number of fundamental empirical and conceptual articles and papers on modern large-scale programs and projects. He has also studied the different types of technological innovation that are manifested in modern society, including small, high-technology firm entrepreneurism, large corporation industrial R&D, and multi-organizational, large-scale programs and projects.

Dr. Horwitch has more recently turned his attention to strategic management and to incorporating technological concerns into the strategic decision-making of the corporation. His current research emphasizes the merging of technology and strategy, the blending of previously distinct modes of technological innovation, and the growing coexistence of multiple and varied approaches for technological development and acquisition by technology-intensive corporations. He is currently completing a book that analyzes the implications of these and other state-of-the-art trends in the strategic management field.

The Editors are deeply grateful to Mel Horwitch for having undertaken the important task of producing such an illuminating and timely contribution to the literature of this field.

— George Bugliarello
A. George Schillinger

Technology in the Modern Corporation

A Strategic Perspective

Managing Corporate Entrepreneurship
New Structures for Implementing Technological Innovation
Robert A. Burgelman

ABSTRACT. *Major changes in the industrial context have put strong pressures on established firms to increase their capacity for technological innovation through internal entrepreneurship. This paper presents a new model of the strategic process, which allows the conceptualization of strategic management challenges associated with such internal entrepreneurship. An assessment framework and an array of design alternatives are also presented to help top management deal with these new challenges. Major implications for the relationships between individuals and large organizations and for the very nature of the corporation of the future are briefly discussed.*

During the 1970s, major segments of American industry — once dominant in world markets — have seen dramatic decline. As Ouchi[1] has observed, the US share of the world market declined by 23% during the 1970s. Not surprisingly, the theme of "Managing Our Way to Economic Decline"[2] has dominated a good deal of the business press during the first half of the 1980s. American management of established firms has been stung by criticisms that their organizations are inadequately innovative, too slow to adapt, inflexible, and short-sighted in their strategic management approaches. The success of *In Search of Excellence*[3] only seems to confirm the intensity with which American managers have been trying to catch up and learn new skills.

This paper examines the current concerns for increased technological innovation through internal entrepreneurship in established firms. The first section of the paper provides an overview of the most recent literature discussing the new industrial context and proposing some new management approaches. The second section presents a new conceptual framework for integrating phenomena regarding internal entrepreneurship in the emerging theory of strategic management. The third section suggests an approach for helping top management deal with the special challenges presented by the strategic management of corporate entrepreneurship. The

Robert A. Burgelman is Associate Professor of Management at the Graduate School of Business, Stanford University. He received his Ph.D. in Management of Organizations from Columbia University in 1980. His research on internal corporate venturing has been published in leading management journals. In 1984, he was the recipient of the Outstanding Paper Award, Division of Business Policy and Planning, Academy of Management. He is co-author of Inside Corporate Innovation *(New York: Free Press [in press]).*

concluding section reflects briefly on the broader implications, which the increased emphasis on internal entrepreneurship will have for the relationships between individuals and large business organizations, and for the very nature of the corporation of the future.

The New Industrial Context for Established Firms

It would, of course, be naive to propose that the relative decline of some segments of American business is solely due to ineptitude on the part of managers of established firms. At least three other major sets of forces should be considered when attempting to diagnose the situation.

First — and perhaps most important — major shifts in relative comparative advantage in factors of production may underly a good deal of the problems encountered by basic American industries. Reich,[4] for instance, has cogently argued that American comparative advantage may lie in more quick-changing, customized product and technology development, rather than in the highly routinized, mature industries, where relative labor cost disadvantages can no longer be overcome by capital improvements. The fact that Japan currently experiences similar pressures as a result of Korean and Taiwanese competition in certain areas may underscore this point.

Second, as the research of Abernathy and Utterback[5] has suggested, some of the setbacks of organizations may be the result of the very logic of technical development: The forces driving the exploitation of existing technological opportunities structurally impede the development of new ones. The classic example is, of course, the American auto industry.[6] Hence, the large aggregations of people and capital represented by the traditional large firms may do well enough — even superbly — when mass production, strict routines, and tightly controlled procedures can be used to attack relatively stable and very large markets. The emphasis of such organizations is, most naturally, on process innovation and improved manufacturing capabilities, not on new product development.

Third, many observers agree that the technological foundations for many of the high-flying industries of the '50s and '60s are now being replaced by new ones — electronics and biotechnology being the clear examples — and require other types of approaches to develop the new entrepreneurial opportunities they offer. Emphasis on new product development and fast-moving strategic positioning and re-positioning are essential here. Not surprisingly, *new* firms have been more adept at performing the entrepreneurial function than established ones. As a result of the "Silicon Valley" effect, entirely new geographical areas are emerging as *loci* of industrial development.

American industry, of course, shows great vigor in these new areas of technology. New firm formation has been rather spectacular — unleashed, in part, by the enormous influx of venture capital after the capital gains tax changes of 1978. Established firms, however, continue to struggle to find new management approaches to return to real growth derived from internal development, rather than from acquisitions.[7]

Some Proposed Solutions

Corresponding to these major shifts in the industrial organizational context and the recognition of significant managerial challenges for established firms, various solutions and approaches have recently been proposed.

Some scholars have focused on the problems of industry maturity and manufacturing competitiveness. Abernathy, Clark and Kantrow[8] have made a useful analysis of the concept of "de-maturity." This refers to the possibility of changing industry dynamics to a point where product technology and innovation can again become tools for creating a competitive advantage. Some recent changes in the automobile industry — GM's Project Saturn, for instance — seem to provide a basis for believing that such an "industrial renaissance" is possible. A major element in these efforts concerns the improved competitiveness in the areas of operations and manufacturing management. As Hayes and Wheelwright[9] have recently suggested, this will require in many cases the full integration of operations and manufacturing considerations in the high-level strategic management of firms.

Other scholars have focused on the broader learning and adaptation capacities of established organizations. Lawrence and Dyer,[10] for instance, present an elaborate discussion of organizational renewal, including recommendations for management-union and management-government relations, geared toward making organizations *both* efficient and innovative, a major challenge, as has been noted earlier. Ouchi[11] has made a strong plea for enlightened "team work" at the organizational level, drawing upon some lessons from the way in which divisionalized firms — the so-called "M-form" organizations — combine hierarchy, market and clan ("cultural") elements in their management processes.

Peters and Waterman[12] have documented some of the approaches used by consistently high-performing US companies. Some of their key recommendations center around the importance of encouraging individuals to experiment, and the capacity of the organization to sustain continuous learning processes. Kanter[13] documents the important role played by middle managers who can initiate both laterally and upwardly to spawn change, in spite of bureaucratic impediments. She describes the behavior of effective change agents as hard-driving individuals with astute views of organizational politics, while Peters and Waterman, in effect, urge top management to give more leeway to such changes by "hanging loose." These would seem, indeed, sensible corrections to a now dated view of a small number of wise top managers controlling, with some precision, the activities of docile and less able followers, and edicting change from above.[14]

The Need for a Theoretical Framework

The natural reaction of companies faced with a new challenge is to seek one-step, well packaged solutions or fixes that look most attractive (and have received wide publicity), and that can be grafted onto the organization with the least trouble, or so it seems. During the 1960s and early '70s, the creation of separate new venture groups seemed to be the answer to the problem of creating truly new businesses for the corporation. This had become a bit of a fad and, when recession struck in the mid-1970s, many such groups were abandoned.[15] Today, the "eight lessons" of Peters and Waterman seem to stand out as the new "quick fix." As *Business Week*[16] recently has observed, however, "excellence" is a transient phenomenon in many cases. Some companies that are no longer excellent didn't continue to adhere, it seems, to the eight lessons. More disturbing, however, some are no longer excellent, even though they *did* adhere to them.

This suggests, perhaps, that even though the quick fixes have significant grains of truth in them, they often fail because they are not based on a solid theoretical framework. Even though less immediately gratifying, it seems useful to work on developing a theoretical framework in the context of which various recommendations and their applicability to particular situations can be examined.

Corporate Entrepreneurship and Strategic Management: A Preliminary Theoretical Framework

As a result of an in-depth field study of the complete process of strategic decision-making regarding internal corporate venturing (ICV),[17] and of reinterpreting the findings of other major field studies,[18] I have proposed a new model of the strategic process. This model is represented in Figure 1.

The new model posits the existence of two fundamentally different processes going on simultaneously in large, complex firms: (1) a process in which the strategic

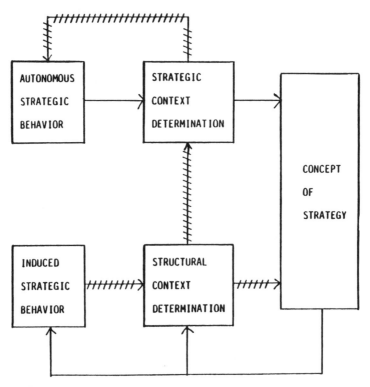

FIGURE 1. A Model of the Strategic Process in Established Firms
Source: (18)

behavior of operational level participants is *induced* by the prevalent concept of strategy of the corporation; and (2) a process in which the *autonomous* strategic behavior of operational level participants forms the basis for amending the firm's concept of strategy. Here is one example of "autonomous" strategic behavior:

> Back in 1980, a manager in Hewlett-Packard Co.'s labs tried to persuade the company's new product people to get into biotechnology. "I was laughed out of the room," says Sam H. Eletr. But venture capitalists didn't laugh. They persuaded Mr. Eletr to quit Hewlett-Packard and staked him to $5.2 million to start a new company. Its product: gene machines, which make DNA, the basic material of the genetic code — and the essential raw material in the burgeoning business of genetic engineering. Now, three years later, Hewlett-Packard has formed a joint venture with Genentech Inc. to develop tools for biotechnology. One product it is considering: gene machines.[18]

The autonomous strategic behavior process corresponds to "corporate entrepreneurship," the elaboration and deepening of the firm's domain of competence and associated opportunity set. The role of internal entrepreneurs is to reveal through *experimentation* with new initiatives what the limits are of the firm's productive capacities. The role of middle and top management is to *select* appropriate entrepreneurial initiatives, and to give them meaning in an enlarged concept of strategy of the firm. Hence strategic "vision" regarding corporate entrepreneurship is fundamentally *ex post*.[20]

The new model provides an explicit theoretical framework from which some of the recommendations proposed by Peters and Waterman[21] can be derived. Identifying the importance of the process of "strategic context" determination, the model provides a further explanation for the key role of middle level managers in the innovation process found in Kanter's studies.[22]

Recently, this model has been further developed[23] to conceptualize emergent strategy-making as a *social learning* process. This provides the basis for integrating the findings of Maidique and Zirger[24] and of Imai *et al.*[25] regarding the new product development process. It also suggests conditions under which important paradigms in organization theory — population ecology,[26] rational adaptation,[27] and "random transformation"[28] — are likely to be helpful in conceptualizing phenomena pertaining to the strategic management process in general.

Managing Internal Entrepreneurship Strategically

From a strategic management perspective, the problem is *how* could corporate management improve its capacity to deal with autonomous strategic behavior, given that, by definition, it does not fit with the current corporate strategy. And, of course, not every new idea or proposal can or should be adopted and developed.

While strategic management associated with the induced strategic behavior loop is based on reasonably well understood planning and cultural influencing techniques, the autonomous strategic behavior loop requires strategic management based on less well understood "experimentation-and-selection" approaches. The model presented earlier proposes, indeed, that the role of top management regarding internal entrepreneurship in large, established firms is primarily one of *strategic recognition*, rather than strategic planning.

An Assessment Framework for Internal Entrepreneurial Proposals

In order to be able to do the selection involved in strategic recognition, top management needs an assessment framework. Such a framework will necessarily comprise multiple dimensions, each of which will be weighted somewhat differently by different top managements. Nevertheless, it seems useful to single out two key dimensions, which should be part of any assessment framework regarding internal entrepreneurial behavior.[29] One of these regards the expected *strategic importance* for corporate development. The other regards the degree to which proposals are related to the core capabilities of the corporation, *i.e.*, their *operational relatedness*.

Assessing strategic importance involves considering the opportunities/threats implied by the entrepreneurial proposal. For instance, in relationship to the example concerning Hewlett-Packard mentioned earlier, the assessment of strategic importance would address the question (among others) whether *not* pursuing the proposal might prevent the corporation from moving into an important new area of electronic instrumentation in the future. This would sharpen the understanding of the trade-offs involved in pursuing strategically related current opportunities, rather than those in the emerging bioelectronics area.

Assessing operational readiness involves examining the implications for current corporate capabilities of the proposal. For instance, in the Hewlett-Packard situation, this might lead to addressing the question whether the capabilities demonstrated by the entrepreneurial initiative reveal new areas which the firm might want to develop further to take advantage of latent technology-based synergies. Bioelectronics could be such an area for a company like Hewlett-Packard.

Determining Appropriate Linkage

The assessment of strategic importance has implications for the degree of *control* corporate management needs to maintain over the new business development. The premise is that firms, like individuals, will want to be able to exert control over those events and circumstances that are likely to affect their strategic positions and thus their freedom to move and pursue their own objectives. This, in turn, has implications for the *administrative linkages* to be established. Examples of administrative linkages concern the way in which strategic objectives are set, resource allocation is managed, and reporting relationships are determined, among others. Administrative linkages can vary from very loose (*e.g.*, reporting relationships only through board members appointed by the parent) to very tight (*e.g.*, reporting relationships fully integrated in corporate hierarchy).

The degree of operational relatedness, on the other hand, has implications for the *efficiency* with which both the new and the existing business can be managed. The premise here is that firms seek to organize their operations in such a way that synergies are maximized while the cost of transactions across internal organizational boundaries are minimized.

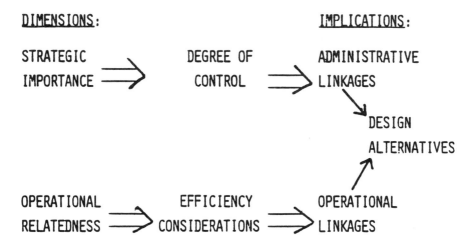

FIGURE 2. Toward an Assessment Framework—Key Dimensions and Their Implications

This, in turn, has implications for the required *operational linkages*. Examples of operational linkages concern, for instance, the ways in which the flows of know-how and information take shape and the degree of integration of workflows, among others. Operational linkages can also vary from loose (*e.g.*, basically independent workflow relations) to quite intense (*e.g.*, mutual adjustment at operational level). Figure 2 shows how the administrative and operational linkages relate to the two key assessment dimensions.

Choosing Design Alternatives

Various combinations of administrative and operational linkages produce different *design alternatives*. These correspond to choices which corporate management has to make regarding the different situations identified in the assessment framework. Figure 3 shows nine such design alternatives.

The design alternatives discussed here are not exhaustive, and the scales for the different dimensions used in the assessment framework remain rudimentary. By the same token, the framework represented in Figure 3 provides a preliminary conceptual underpinning for a number of practices encountered in today's business environment.[30]

1. *Direct Integration*. High strategic importance and operational relatedness require strong administrative and operational linkages. This means, in fact, the need to integrate the new business directly into the mainstream of the corporation. Such integration must anticipate internal resistance for reasons well documented in the organizational change literature. The role of "champions" knowing the workings of the current system well are likely to be important in such situations. The need for direct integration is perhaps most likely to occur in fairly highly integrated firms, where radical changes in product concept and/or in process technologies could threaten the overall strategic position of the firm.[31]

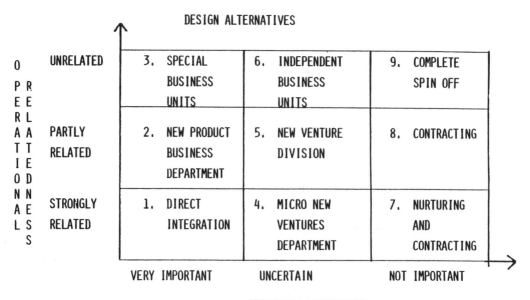

FIGURE 3. Organization Designs for Corporate Entrepreneurship
Source: (29)

2. *New Product/Business Department.* High strategic importance and partial operational relatedness require a combination of strong administrative and medium strong operational linkages. This may be achieved by creating a separate department around an entrepreneurial project in that part (division or group) of the operating system where potential for sharing capabilities and skills is significant. Corporate management should monitor the strategic development of the project in substantive terms, and not allow it to be folded (and "buried") into the overall strategic planning of that division or group.[32]

3. *Special Business Units.* High strategic importance and low operational relatedness may require the creation of specially dedicated new business units. Strong administrative linkages are necessary to ensure the attainment of explicit strategic objectives within specific time horizons throughout the development process. It will be often necessary to combine and integrate some of these business units into a new operating division in the corporate structure, later on.[33]

4. *Micro New Ventures Department.* Uncertain strategic importance and high operational relatedness seem typical for the "peripheral" projects which are likely to emerge in the operating division on a rather continuous basis. For such projects, administrative linkages should be loose. The venture manager should be allowed to develop a strategy within budget and time constraints, but otherwise would not be limited by current divisional or even corporate level strategies. Operational linkages should be strong to take advantage of the existing capabilities and skills and to facilitate transferring back newly developed ones. Norman Fast[34] has discussed a "micro" new ventures division design which would seem to fit the conditions specified here.

5. *New Venture Division.* This design is proposed for situations of maximum ambiguity in the assessment framework.[35] In the light of these ambiguities, top management is likely to want a certain degree of direct control over activities which may turn out to be of strategic importance for corporate development. Hence, they will want to keep them *internal*, at least until greater clarity concerning their strategic importance is reached. But top management is also likely to want to protect the efficiency of the operating system. Hence, they will want to keep the new venture activities *separate*, at least until their degree of operational relatedness becomes clearer. The NVD design has the potential to satisfy both of these top management concerns.

    The NVD may serve best as a "nucleation" function.[35] It provides a fluid internal environment for projects with the potential to create major new business thrusts for the corporation, but of which the strategic importance remains to be determined as the development process unfolds. Administrative' linkages should be fairly loose. Middle-level managers supervising a few ventures are expected to develop "middle range" strategies for new fields of business: bringing together projects which may exist in various parts of the corporation, and/or which can be acquired externally, and integrating these with some of the venture projects they supervise to build sizeable new businesses. Operational linkages should also be fairly loose — yet be sufficiently developed to facilitate transferring back and forth relevant know-how and information concerning capabilities and skills. Long-time horizons — eight to 12 years — are necessary, but ventures should not be allowed to languish. High-quality middle-level managers are crucial to make this design work.

6. *Independent Business Units.* Uncertain strategic importance and negligible operational relatedness may make external venture arrangements attractive. Different degrees of controlling ownership with correspondingly strong board representation may provide corporate management with an acceptable level of strategic control.[37]

7. *Nurturing Plus Contracting.* In some cases, an entrepreneurial proposal may be considered unimportant for the firm's corporate development strategy, yet be strongly related to its operational capabilities and skills. Such ventures will typically address "interstices" in the market,[38] which may be too small for the company to serve profitably, but which offer opportunities for a small business. Top management may want to help such entrepreneurs spin off from the corporation, and may, in fact, help the entrepreneur set up his or her business. The present company could also decide to obtain a minority participation in the new business. This provides a known, and most likely, friendly competitor in those interstices, keeping out others. There may be a basis for long-term contracting relationships in which the corporation can profitably supply the entrepreneur with some of its excess capabilities and skills. Strong operational linkages related to these contracts may facilitate transfer of new or improved skills developed by the entrepreneur.[39]

8. *Contracting.* The possibilities for nurturing would seem to diminish as the required capabilities and skills of the new business are less related. Yet there may still be opportunities for profitable contracting arrangements, and for

learning about new or improved capabilities and skills through some forms of operational linkages.

9. *Complete Spin Off.* If strategic importance and operational relatedness are both low, complete spin off will be most appropriate. A decision based on a careful assessment of both dimensions is likely to lead to a well founded decision from the perception of both the corporation and the internal entrepreneur.

Implementing Design Alternatives

In order to implement designs for corporate entrepreneurship effectively, three major issues and potential problems need to be further considered. First, corporate management and the internal entrepreneur should view the assessment framework as a tool to clarify—at a particular moment in time—their community of interests and interdependencies, and to structure a non-zero sum game.

Second, corporate management must establish measurement and reward systems which are capable of accommodating the different incentive requirements of different designs.

Third, as the development process unfolds, new information may modify the perceived strategic importance and operational relatedness, which may require a renegotiation of the organization design.

To deal effectively with the implementation issues and potential problems, corporate management must recognize internal entrepreneurs as "strategists," perhaps even *encourage* them to think/act as such. This is necessary, because the stability of the relationship will be dependent upon both parties feeling that they have achieved their individual interests to the greatest extent, given the structure of the situation. On the part of corporate management, this implies attempts to appropriate benefits from the entrepreneurial endeavor, but only to the extent that they can provide the entrepreneur with the opportunity to be more successful than he or she would be going it alone. This, in turn, requires simultaneously generous policies to help internal entrepreneurs, based on a sound assessment of their proposals, and unequivocal determination to protect proprietary corporate capabilities and skills vigorously.[40]

Conclusion:
A New Organizational Revolution in the Making?

Until recently, the Schumpeterian distinction between entrepreneurial and administrated ("bureaucratic") economic activity could be considered adequate. In the light of the turbulence of recent industrial developments, however, this distinction seems to lose much of its relevance. Large, established corporations are confronted with the problem of maintaining their growth, if not their existence, by exploiting to the fullest the unique resource combinations they have assembled.

Increasingly there is an awareness that internal entrepreneurs are necessary for firms to achieve this. Because, like the external entrepreneur, the internal entrepreneur enacts new opportunities and drives the development of new resource combinations or recombinations. As a result, new forms of economic organization—a broader array of arrangements—seems necessary.

This, in turn, requires a theory of the firm based on a more nuanced view of the role of hierarchies, contracts and markets. The conceptual foundations of this are currently being laid in such fields as the economics of internal organization and information, agency theory, the theory of legal contracts, and theories of organization design and change.

The outlines of a strategic management theory of corporate entrepreneurship are still dim. But I believe that it will be grounded in increased understanding of the evolutionary processes of organizational learning. In these evolutionary organizational learning processes, entrepreneural *individuals* at operational and middle levels will play an increasingly important role. There exists some evidence of the fact that such individuals elaborate the organization's capabilities and enact the new opportunities which are associated with the elaboration efforts. In a very important sense, they help their organizations to enlarge and embroider their "knitting," rather than just sticking to the existing knitting.

The challenge for American managers will be to integrate new theoretical insights quickly, as they become available. This challenge is real, because the Japanese (and perhaps others as well) are already aware of the need to do so.[41]

Individualism and Big Business: A New Beginning

This leads to another theme. The inquiry into the nature of corporate entrepreneurship provides the basis for a rather optimistic view. But, at the same time, it suggests a tremendous challenge for top management of established firms.

Almost continuously, established firms hire from the best and brightest graduates the nation's educational system has to offer. Systematic surveys (supported by one's limited but direct contact with students) seem to suggest that a significant number of these young people have entrepreneurial aspirations, and are looking for something more than the job security traditionally offered by large, established firms. On the one hand, this creates a necessity for dramatic changes in the management practices of large, established firms, if they want to be able to compete with glittering new firms for entrepreneurial talent. On the other hand, it suggests the existence of an enormous potential for corporate entrepreneurship ready to exert itself and to be channeled into directions beneficial to both the individual and the firm.

The existence of this potential, it is perhaps worth noting, was proposed more than 20 years ago by Leonard R. Sayles and others, who critically examined the foundations for the widely asserted contradiction between "individualism" and "big business," and found them lacking.[42] Now, it would seem the times are ripe for a new integration of individualism and big business through strategies for corporate entrepreneurship.

One should, therefore, perhaps be cautious with respect to recommendations, currently fashionable, to create a homogenous and overly integrative "corporate culture." The challenge for established firms, it would seem, is not to be either well organized and to act in unison, or to be creative and entrepreneurial. The real challenge is to be able to live with the tensions generated by both. This will require top management to secure the exploitation of existing opportunities to the fullest (because only relatively few will be available); the generation of entirely new opportunities (because today's success is no guarantee of tomorrow's); and the balancing of opportunity exploitation and generation over time (because resources are limited). Strategic management will have to accomplish all these concerns simultaneously and virtually continuously.

The Corporation of the Future

The last theme, then, concerns the evolving nature of the established firm. The developments currently crystalizing in American business may quite possibly indicate an epochal change. This change may well be of the same magnitude as the one that occurred during the first quarter of the 20th century, which led to the organizational innovation represented by the "divisionalized firm," brilliantly documented in Alfred D. Chandler's landmark study on strategy and structure.[43]

The new wave of organizational innovations involves, as noted earlier, new types of arrangements between individuals and corporations. It is likely to continue to produce new organizational forms, spanning the entire range of combinations of markets and hierarchies.[44] As noted, this will involve complex, sometimes protracted *negotiation processes* between individual and corporate actors. Such negotiation processes will most likely be an increasingly pervasive aspect of corporate life, and an important mechanism for facilitating the new integration of individualism and big business through corporate entrepreneurship.

Acknowledgments

Support from the Strategic Management Program of Stanford University's Graduate School of Business is gratefully acknowledged. Parts of the introduction and conclusion of this paper are based on R.A. Burgelman and L.R. Sayles, *Inside Corporate Innovation: Strategy, Structure, and Managerial Skills* (New York: Free Press, in press).

Notes and References

1. Ouchi points out that the tables had already started turning in the 1960s, when American industry lost 16% of its share of world markets, while another 23% was lost during the 1970s. See William Ouchi, *The M-Form Society* (Reading, MA: Addison-Wesley, 1984), p. 3.
2. Robert Hayes and William Abernathy, "Managing Our Way to Economic Decline," *Harvard Business Review*, July–August 1980.
3. T. Peters and R. Waterman, *In Search of Excellence* (New York: Harper and Row, 1982).
4. Robert Reich, *The New American Frontier* (New York: Times Books, 1983).
5. W. Abernathy and J. Utterback, "Patterns of Industrial Innovation," *Technology Review—Innovation* (1976).
6. William Abernathy, *The Productivity Dilemma* (Baltimore: Johns Hopkins University Press, 1978).
7. For some examples of the problems associated with acquisitions, see: "Raytheon Is Among Companies Regretting High-Tech Mergers," *The Wall Street Journal*, September 10, 1984. For an example of successful acquisition strategies, see: "Gould Reshapes Itself into High-Tech Outfit Amid Much Turmoil," *The Wall Street Journal*, October 10, 1984.
8. W. Abernathy, K. Clark and A. Kantrow, *Industrial Renaissance* (New York: Basic Books, 1983).
9. Robert Hayes and Steven Wheelwright, *Regaining Our Competitive Edge* (New York: Wiley, 1984).
10. Paul Lawrence and Davis Dyer, *Renewing American Industry* (New York: Free Press, 1983).
11. W. Ouchi, *op. cit.*
12. T. Peter and R. Waterman, *op. cit.*
13. R. Kanter, *The Change Masters* (New York: Basic Books, 1983).
14. Katherine D. Fishman, for instance, describes IBM's Tom Watson's understandable frustration at not being able to get his extraordinary organization to turn out a large computer to compete with Control Data's big

machines. See Katherine D. Fishman, *The Computer Establishment* (New York: Harper and Row, 1981).

15. The abandonment of many new venture divisions has been documented by Norman Fast, *The Rise and Fall of New Venture Divisions* (Ann Arbor, MI: UMI Research Press, 1979).

16. "Oops!" *Business Week*, November 8, 1984.

17. R.A. Burgelman, "A Process Model of Internal Corporate Venturing in the Diversified Major Firm," *Administrative Science Quarterly*, June 1983.

18. R.A. Burgelman, "A Model of the Interaction of Strategic Behavior, Corporate Context, and the Concept of Strategy," *Academy of Management Review*, January 1983.

19. "After Slow Start, Gene Machines Approach a Period of Fast Growth and Steady Profits," *The Wall Street Journal*, December 13, 1983.

20. R.A. Burgelman, "Corporate Entrepreneurship and Strategic Management: Insights from a Process Study," *Management Science*, December 1983.

21. T. Peters and R. Waterman, *op. cit.*

22. R. Kanter, *op. cit.*

23. R.A. Burgelman, "Strategy-Making and Evolutionary Theory: Towards a Capabilities-Based Perspective," Research Paper Series #755, Graduate School of Business, Stanford University, 1984.

24. M. Maidique and B.J. Zirger, "The Success-Failure Cycle in New Product Development," Working Paper, School of Industrial Engineering and Engineering Management, Stanford University, 1984.

25. K. Imai, I. Nonaka and H. Takeuchi, "Managing the New Product Development Process: How Japanese Companies Learn and Unlearn," Discussion Paper no. 118, Hitotsubashi University, Japan, 1984.

26. M. Hanan and J. Freeman, "Structural Inertia and Organizational Change," *American Sociological Review*, April 1984.

27. J. Pfeffer and G. Salancik, *The External Control of Organizations: A Resource Dependence Perspective* (New York: Harper and Row, 1978).

28. J. March, "Footnotes on Organizational Change," *Administrative Science Quarterly*, December 1981.

29. R.A. Burgelman, "Designs for Corporate Entrepreneurship in Established Firms," *California Management Review*, Spring 1984.

30. For a complementary discussion of some of these new approaches, see: E.B. Roberts, "New Ventures for Corporate Growth," *Harvard Business Review*, July–August 1980.

31. An example of the need for direct integration is documented by Twiss's account of the development of "float glass" at Pilkington Glass Ltd. See B. Twiss, *Managing Technological Innovation* (London: Longman, 1980).

32. An example where the proposed approach might have been useful is provided by one of the major diversified automotive supplier's handling of electronic fuel injection development. In spite of the fact that they had the right technology, there was strong resistance from the firm's automotive group management level which did not support the development. Only after a new group level manager took charge of the strategic management of the project and brought in additional operational capabilities and skills did the project take off. See Bendix Corporation (A) (9-378-257), HBS Case Services, Harvard Business School, Boston.

33. IBM's use of the Special Business Unit design to enter the personal computer business is an example. See "Meet the New Lean, Mean IBM," *Fortune*, June 13, 1983, p. 78.

34. N.D. Fast, *The Rise and Fall of Corporate New Venture Divisions* (Ann Arbor: U.M.I. Research Press, 1979).

35. R.A. Burgelman, "Managing the New Venture Division: Research Findings and Implications for Strategic Management," *Strategic Management Journal*, January–March 1985.

36. See: "Allied Unit, Free of Red Tape, Seeks to Develop Orphan Technologies," *The Wall Street Journal*, September 10, 1984.

37. IBM's use of Independent Business Units is one example where the corporation keeps complete ownership. See *Fortune, op. cit.* An example of joint ownership is provided by the way that the Bank of America has organized its Venture-Capital Business. See "Despite Greater Risks, More Banks Turn to Venture-Capital Business," *The Wall Street Journal*, November 28, 1983.

38. For a discussion of the concept of "interstice," see E.T. Penrose, *The Theory of the Growth of the Firm* (Oxford: Blackwell, 1968).

39. See: "Tektronix New-Venture Subsidiary Brings Benefits to Parent, Spinoffs," *The Wall Street Journal*, September 18, 1984.

40. For an account of some examples, see "Spinoffs Mount in Silicon Valley," *The New York Times*, January 3, 1984.

41. A good indicator of this is the emphasis on the internal corporate ventures, and on the need for new approaches to strategic management in large, established firms currently emphasized by the Japanese. See: "Business Management in the New Industrial Revolution," White Paper 1983, Japan Committee for Economic Development, pp. 14–15.

42. L.R. Sayles, *Individualism and Big Business* (New York: McGraw-Hill, 1964).

43. A.D. Chandler, *Strategy and Structure* (Cambridge, MA: The MIT Press, 1962).

44. O.E. Williamson, *Markets and Hierarchies* (New York: Free Press, 1975).

Technological Innovation and Interdependence

A Challenge for the Large, Complex Firm

Yves Doz, Reinhard Angelmar and C.K. Prahalad

ABSTRACT. *Faced with accelerating change in their technological environment, managers of large, complex firms must ensure that relevant new technologies are developed and utilized for the rejuvenation of existing and the creation of new businesses. Responsibility for managing this process has rested traditionally with existing research and development units. Growing dissatisfaction with this solution has led to new approaches for innovation, such as internal venturing, which attempt to emulate small, entrepreneurial companies. In this article, the authors argue that all approaches to innovation that remain confined to individual organizational units, be they existing or especially created, lead to suboptimal results when the technologies involved have implications for several business units. They then discuss a number of organizational capabilities that are necessary to differentiate innovative activities from on-going operations, and yet — at the same time — allow large, complex firms to exploit their unique advantages by integrating their new and existing activities. Administrative mechanisms available to top management for shaping the organizational context are discussed next. Finally, the authors present two illustrative cases from their research.*

Most large, complex firms carry out R&D activities, both in central research establishments and in the different operating divisions. Under the guidance of group and divisional management, these R&D units are charged with the mission of ensuring the discovery and development of new technologies, the exploitation of which is entrusted to the non-R&D parts or the operating divisions.

The main complaint in companies with large, well-funded R&D establishments

Yves Doz is Associate Professor of Business Policy at INSEAD. He is the author of two books and a number of articles on multinational management, based on an extensive research program in a score of multinational companies. His current research interests focus on the management of innovation in large, complex, multinational firms.

Reinhard Angelmar is Associate Professor of Marketing at INSEAD. He was educated at the Hochschule für Welthandel in Vienna, Austria (Diplomkaufmann, 1968), and at Northwestern University, Evanston, Illinois (MBA, 1971; Ph.D., 1976). His research and publications have been in the areas of philosophy of science, distribution, governmental regulation, and innovation.

C.K. Prahalad is Associate Professor of Policy and Control at the University of Michigan. His research focuses on competition in global industries and on strategies for emerging industries and complex innovations. He is the author of several articles on strategic management in multinational companies.

is that they seem to have difficulty in moving quickly on new innovations, and in being sufficiently sensitive to market needs. While speed is not always a critical factor, it may become so as technological change accelerates. For example, genetic engineering may remove long-term patent protection, and transform the climate in the pharmaceutical industry into a rat race. Similarly, speed is essential in consumer electronics as product life-cycles shorten and as the industry becomes global.[1] Excessive "technology push," the other major shortcoming of firms with large research establishments, may lead these companies to develop mistargeted technologies and products for which there is no demand, or in which there is no basis for sustained competitive advantage.

These observations are frequently generalized by executives and academics alike to suggest that large firms suffer from an intrinsic disadvantage in innovating. Several considerations underlie this suggestion. To carry out complex, interrelated tasks, large firms develop formal structures which fragment these tasks into elements that can be performed by individuals, and integrate these elements through formal hierarchies and rules. The bureaucracy that results, the power plays that surround the rules, and the often fragile authority of key managers discourage innovation and risk-taking. This has been variously described as "segmentalist" behavior[2] and bureaucratic "resistance to change".[3] Analyses of resource allocation processes in large firms confirm that view.[4] The larger and more diversified firms become, the more their management systems evolve toward a logic of control and guidance, and away from a logic of entrepreneurship and variety creation; the more efficient management becomes, the more the on-going takes precedence over developing the new. Managers see this as a serious problem.

Emulation of Small, Entrepreneurial Companies

Small entrepreneurial firms, often created by innovators who left big firms, have been a main motor in the exploitation of technological progress. These firms operate in a free market, to which they have to be very sensitive, away from hierarchical constraints and safety nets, under the drive of an entrepreneur. They are usually characterized by a great freedom to act, considerable financial incentives to the entrepreneurs, a high willingness to take risks, and the dedication of a small team toward one single project around a charismatic technical leader who drives the effort. These characteristics are all believed to allow more innovations and new business opportunities to be pursued faster, and often with better success, than do the traditional R&D centers of major firms.

Informal group organization in the entrepreneurial firms with fluid, ill-defined structures, group processes, and flat hierarchies allow these entrepreneurial firms to tackle the task uncertainties and interdependencies better than more formal structures.[5] Piqued by the success of these small, entrepreneurial firms and following the examples of companies such as 3M and Hewlett-Packard, large firms have taken to emulating small ones, and the "small is beautiful" culture has often come to pervade them. These firms institutionalized the arrangements as "entrepreneurial subsidiaries," "skunkworks," "independent product teams," "new venture groups," and "internal corporate ventures."[6] Their common concept is to focus innovative efforts in small, self-contained, autonomous teams directed toward specific new products and businesses, either throughout the corporation (3M, Hewlett-Packard) or selectively via a new venture group overseeing internal corporate ventures (the companies analyzed by Fast[7] and Burgelman[8]). These arrangements became common practice in the US during the 1970s, following early reports of their success at 3M, Owens Illinois, and DuPont.[9] In the early 1980s, the growing preoccupation with the rejuvenation of US industry made these common wisdom.[10]

Yet recent research (Fast, 1978; Burgelman, 1980, 1985) has pointed out some shortcomings of internal venturing.[11] First, new ventures may find it difficult to obtain the right type of managers and other key personnel; personal profiles, career paths and reward systems may conflict between the core businesses and the new independent efforts. Second, competition takes place within large firms for resources and for top management attention, and the new ventures may be neglected.[12] Third, the interests of venture managers (or, in some cases, partners) are likely to conflict with those of the corporate parent.[13]

Finally—and most importantly—new ventures do not always allow the easy exploitation of valuable potential interdependencies between the core businesses (and their technologies) and the new ventures. It is difficult for the independent ventures to tap into the corporate competencies and resources, because their needs conflict with other units' operating priorities, and control systems tend to reinforce —rather than transcend—organizational boundaries.

Technological Innovation and Interdependence

The same new technologies may simultaneously affect different businesses, but in different ways, either because they can be used by several of them (*e.g.*, laser technology at Philips, or digital signaling equipment at EMI), be instrumental in their convergence (*e.g.*, local area networks for office products), or provide a common core technology to several businesses (*e.g.*, microelectronics, composite materials, or genetic engineering). Innovative applications may also require the combinations of innovations into complex systems (*e.g.*, fiber optics communications). Both core technologies and system technologies create relatedness across the businesses they affect.

Core and system technologies cutting across existing businesses for the scientific bases or market applications create difficulties both for the small firm emulation and the traditional approaches to managing innovation in large, complex firms.

While new ventures and similar organizational arrangements allow speedy entrepreneurial development of technologies, they also tend to suffer from isolation and face difficulties when their results have to be integrated into existing businesses, particularly when such effort must serve the somewhat divergent needs of multiple businesses. Basically, the small-company approach results in an underutilization of the potential synergies of large, complex firms.

Assigning responsibilities for new technologies to existing business units may have a similar effect. The emphasis on product-market focus that has characterized much of the recent research and practice on corporate planning (via strategic business unit [SBU] and portfolio concepts) essentially ignores interdependencies across businesses and markets. No single unit may provide a breadth of view and depth of commitment sufficient to consider the various potential applications and pursue them successfully. Thus, entrusting an existing business unit with the responsibility of developing the new technology may lead to a narrow focus or to marginal commitment, if the technology is not a critical priority for the unit involved. Ignoring interdependencies through an excessive emphasis on individual product-market applications weakens a firm's technological basis and may result in lost markets.[14]

In contrast with the product-market focus of many large Western companies, many Japanese companies consider core technologies as the permanent basis of their business and specific application areas as transient opportunities.[15] This has enabled them to build up strong technological advantages over their competitors. Some Western companies have recently reorganized in order to benefit from cross-unit dependencies. For example, Hewlett-Packard, typically cited as an example of a large company consisting of a collection of independently managed business units, recently reorganized in order to allow exploitation of market and customer interdependencies.

Differentiation and Interdependence: Shifting Priorities

In sum, *for core and system technologies, both differentiation from and interdependence with existing businesses are needed.* Entrepreneurial ventures provide for differentiation, but make integration difficult, while integration into an existing division may neither allow response to needs from multiple units nor provide a fast and strong enough response to new technologies.

Needs for differentiation and benefits from interdependence may shift over time continuously. This is seen in Figure 1. When new technologies are only emerging, interdependencies may be low, and research efforts or new ventures may have a "listening post" or "insurance" function (what if this new technology suddenly takes off and affects our core businesses?). Later on, while differentiation may remain important, interdependencies with operating businesses (*e.g.*, to specify the parameters of the innovation as a function of possible applications) may become much more important. Also, to succeed, the new innovation may have to draw on resources and competencies scattered in various established organizational units. Once the R&D effort is being carried out, integration may predominate for concrete implementation of the innovation, particularly where it involves process changes of some significance in manufacturing and marketing. Product innovation is easier to fold back into a well-established operation than process or system innovation, which calls for the creation, transfer and application of new practical knowledge on actual tasks.

So far, we have argued that conventional organizational options suffer from intrinsic limitations that make them less and less capable of coping with the technological demands put on large, complex firms whose businesses are both diverse and related. We suggested that the growing emphasis on core and system technologies creates needs for high levels of differentiation between innovative and operational activities, and also calls for strong capabilities to manage the interdependencies between them. The growing need for speed in technology and product development

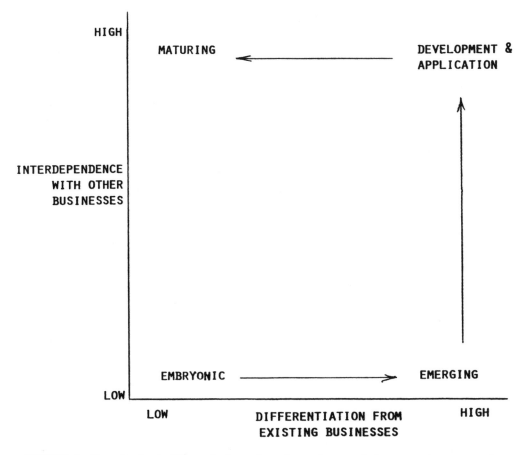

FIGURE 1. Hypothesized differentiation—interdependence mix in managing core technology innovation over time.

further compounds the problems by imposing severe time limits on coordination processes.

The remainder of this paper first details the capabilities required of large, complex firms to achieve core technology and system innovation and then outlines some possible approaches to developing such capabilities, based on our study of innovation processes within selected firms.[16]

Managing Differentiation and Interdependence: The Required Capabilities

The Need for Multiple Perspectives

To jointly recognize and assess the needs for interdependence and differentiation, organization processes must allow the company to be viewed by its members from several perspectives. As core and system technologies come to predominate, integrative perspectives on these technologies are increasingly required to counter the fragmentation pressures implicit in product-market planning. An electronics company, for instance, can be seen as a set of different portfolios, each portfolio vision being useful for certain purposes, but not all. For some purposes, the company is a portfolio of core technologies, each with multiple business and system applications. For other purposes, a portfolio of strategic business units may predominate, or a portfolio of "strategic families".[17] For others, yet other visions of a portfolio – such as application engineering capabilities, manufacturing skills, or market access investments – may alternatively or jointly be useful.

Such multiple perspectives can be maintained in various ways. First, information systems may be multifocal rather than unidimensional, and sustain multiple visions of the firm's activities. For instance, it should be possible to consider investments in core technologies, or in distribution, independent of specific business units, which – on their own – may not see it as in their interests. This calls for complex information processing capabilities for the firm, both internally between the activities of its various sub-units, and externally *vis-a-vis* its environment. Nippon Electric (NEC), for instance, has evolved a complex structure of coordinating committees that overlap its organizational units and allow the maintenance of a multi-unit perspective on relevant issues.[18]

Flexible Resource Allocation Channels

To help sustain multiple perspectives and to make them sufficiently important for managers, resources must flow in various ways. Until recently, for instance, Matsushita's business units could freely reinvest – on their own – about 40% of their cash flow. While this supported entrepreneurship and innovation at business level, it made the funding of major corporate efforts – such as new technology development – difficult. In particular, Matsushita found itself lagging behind its major competitors in microelectronics, which were fast becoming a critical core technology for all its businesses. In the early 1980s, Matsushita recentralized almost all key resource allocation decisions, and thus limited the autonomy of the business units. Autonomous investment strategies were no longer to be pursued by product departments and divisions.[19]

Conversely, the well-known 3M sponsorship policies – whereby internal innovators can knock on multiple doors to get funded – or Texas Instruments' "wild hare" programs correspond to a concern for increasing variety by encouraging "autonomous" strategic behavior.[20] Although the amounts are often small, they do allow the initial development of ideas that will make later assessments, the commitment of resources, or the decision to end the project easier.

Our argument is that companies need both approaches to resource allocation: the ability to focus resources from multiple units toward large-scale corporate projects for core technologies (such as Matsushita's investments in microelectronics), and also the ability to encourage smaller-scale entrepreneurial efforts.

Several of the large companies analyzed in our research experienced resource allocation difficulties for innovative products. Essentially, they fell into a resource allocation trap. The inertia and stability of their large research and development establishment only allowed for marginal changes to the pattern of resource allocation to innovative projects. Researchers also developed a culture whereby large resource allocation shifts, in what they perceived to be a zero-sum game within a stable overall budget, were not sought. Social norms of belonging and balance made active competition for resources difficult to accept. Innovators and researchers could opt out of the usual marginal resource reallocation patterns, and go for big commitments. But, since these were big, they were treated essentially as other major investments (*e.g.*, plant capacity) and had to be backed up by extensive analysis, forecasts, and quantitative data.

Faced with the dilemma of accepting an incremental approach or providing a false sense of certainty to their projects, innovators reacted as a function of their own idiosyncrasies and backgrounds. Scientists resigned themselves to marginal increases in resources, and "business" innovators (*e.g.*, product champions coming from marketing) dressed up their projects with optimistic numbers. People with successful track records went for incremental increases, while entrepreneurs who had already failed in the past had little to lose and went for bigger and riskier options. Over time, both approaches were likely to lead to failures—of omission, in the first case; of commission, in the second—which then deterred further entrepreneurship around new projects. Perceived risks—were they only to lose face—were too high.

The Need to Explicitly Manage Personal Risks and Rewards

Large, complex firms may have to manage personal risks explicitly, so that risks can be purposefully concentrated or spread out. In a study of innovation in the electronics industry, Schwartz noted the importance of "factoring" risks, *i.e.*, of breaking risks down into well-defined components that can be accepted by the individuals.[21] Schwartz argues that planning and reward processes may be used both to factor the risks and to make them acceptable to individuals. The balance between risk-concentration and risk-sharing ought to vary with the nature of the innovation. While concentrating risks on a key individual, who takes them as a personal challenge (*e.g.*, "Don" Estridge at the start of the IBM personal computer or Tom West in Kidder's account of a project at Data General), makes sense for a new venture or a discrete project; core or system technology projects call for multiple contributors, and risks cannot be all assumed by any of them.[22] Yet risk-taking is highly personal, and a group may shy away from bold initiatives, or find it difficult to reach a consensus on the acceptable level of risk. Therefore, the factoring of risks into manageable, acceptable subsets and their explicit allocation to individuals are critical requirements for the large, complex firms.

Rewards raise parallel issues. While "hero-projects" of much visibility to corporate managements and criticality to the firms usually attract significant rewards to their champions and sponsors (according to the usual roles in the innovation processes described, for instance, by Maidique) large companies too often tend to be unresponsive to entrepreneurial performance.[23] Exceptional entrepreneurship may go unrewarded, or, worse, the innovator may attract more criticism and bad feeling from "rocking the boat" than praise for being entrepreneurial, even when he or she succeeds.

Flexible Modes of Managing People

Management of the routine activities of large, complex firms typically relies on hierarchy as a means of coordinating the efforts of individuals and groups. Prescriptions for increasing innovativeness typically point out the inappropriateness of hierarchies and suggest other modes of regulations. Three alternatives are: 1) market mechanisms; 2) organizational culture; and 3) networks.

Market Mechanisms. Conventional internal venturing processes with their objectives to stimulate the conditions of start-up companies can be summarized as attempts to bring market mechanisms back into the big firm, and substitute these for the more structured and more stable mechanisms that operate in the labor market. Equity positions, stock incentives, etc., all support that direction. They may work well when the venture is to become a true, independent spin-off, and when the main aim of the parent company is to provide genuine entreprenurial stimulation and make capital gains when the venture goes public. When, however, independent units may be only temporary (*e.g.*, since their product is closely related to that of the parent), reliance on strong financial incentives and market mechanisms may considerably complicate the reintegration process. Memorex, for instance, faltered when it tried to reintegrate its "entrepreneurial subsidiaries" into the fold of a single multiproduct "Memorex Equipment Group."[24] Conversely, in its "Independent Business Units," IBM insisted that usual corporate employment policies be applied, and the personal incentives to managers were relatively modest. While this may have created some tensions (in particular, between IBM employees, who remained salaried and their subcontractors, who sometimes made a fortune from supplying IBM's PC venture), it eased the subsequent reintegration of some IBUs (such as the personal computers) into IBM and the mobility of personnel between the main business and the IBUs. Similarly, IBM has extended only limited financial rewards to its innovators and product champions.

Organizational Culture. Companies such as IBM and 3M have relied more on a cultural approach toward differentiation, which also makes interdependence easier to achieve. Its premise is that, when the individual interests of the members of the organization (the common interests of its members in contributing to the organization) are aligned closely enough to reach a substantial overlap, many of the problems of large organizations are much attenuated, in particular, parochialism and narrow subgoals.[25] Such an approach has been labeled variously as the building of "clans," a "communal" approach, or a corporate culture or corporate identity approach.[26] These various definitions are usually rooted in some reintegration of certain traits of Japanese management practice, but are also logically derived from an examination of corporate management tools and the regulation of relationships between corporate and subunit management.[27]

While the "clan" approach has many advantages, and some evidence in its favor (*e.g.*, Kanter's[28] descriptions of the features of "integrative companies," or Peters and Waterman's[29] descriptions of "excellent" companies), it still faces some limits. First, it may apply mostly to small companies where community spirit and high commitment may revolve around single founder-entrepreneurs. In large companies, attempts to institutionalize a clan approach to innovation run the risk of degenerating into the mechanical replication of innovative conditions that once succeeded, rather than maintaining the spirit of true innovation. (Jelinek's analysis of Texas Instruments, although it purports to describe a highly innovative company, describes a company suffering from this syndrome.[30] A casual observation of Texas Instruments' track record with new business development suggests that, while it could codify, institutionalize and replicate the implicit approach that made it successful in semiconductors, the company found it difficult to adjust to tasks and businesses that also required organizational innovation (*e.g.*, consumer products). In other words, small clans exist more easily than large ones, and the "clan" approach may best apply to specific projects, (*e.g.*, the product development team described by Kidder, rather than the whole of Data General). Maintaining a "clan" spirit in a large firm—no matter of which nationality—may be difficult unless the spirit of its founder remains strong (IBM or Matsushita in the 1960s). The rapid evolution of Apple Computers from a small clan to a large firm with multiple divisions, and the human attrition that accompanied it testify to the difficulty of maintaining a clan approach in a large, fast-growing firm.[31]

Second, a clan approach may limit the extent of differentiation and entrepreneurship, and lead more to a "village" approach (people have to coexist, but cooperate only to a limited effect) or a "family" approach (where the common identity comes from a common past, rather than a shared future). In such cases, differentiation often remains insufficient, while integration may be lacking in precision. Mediocre decisions and difficulties in implementation may result. Finally, even if it remains suitable, a clan approach is not available to all companies; it is built over time and rooted in a firm's history. It cannot be built rapidly from a different corporate culture or identity.

Networks. A third approach has sometimes been labeled "networks." Networks can process information in multiple directions, and allow for fluid configuration of differentiation and integration. They are usually based on a complex web of perceived material obligations between members of the organization.[32] By facilitating the exchange of information and the provision of support within the organization, they may provide the opportunity for innovation by bringing together different logics and data (a frequent condition for creativity and innovation), encouraging actual innovative behavior by providing channels for business consensus, and providing specific support to the innovation. Networks facilitate both the flow of new technology[33] and the development of innovation efforts.

Networks do not function on their own, however. They are rooted in specific ways of managing and providing incentives for individuals in rotations of people of a kind that may not be functional for R&D personnel and, in particular, characteristic of the exchanges between them.[34] They may not overcome the absence of trust created by a small number of critical transactions. Networks, like the other three models of regulation of the management of innovation, have advantages and disadvantages that make them more or less appropriate to various types of innovation.

While each mode of managing innovators (the conventional hierarchy of large companies, market mechanisms, clan cultures, and network relationships) possesses limits, they point toward the possibility of blending them in mixed fashions to vary the degree of differentiation and interdependence between the innovating and the operating activities. Our detailed analysis of organizational processes surrounding innovation parallels some broader studies of organizational adaptation.[35]

Flexibility Over Time

As suggested in the beginning of this paper, the needs for differentiation and inter-dependence shift over time. For instance, personal computers have evolved from being stand-alone "toys" for the hobbyist to the home user, to desk top units for the professional and the manager, and now as a substitute for terminals and parts of interconnected networks.

Organizations, contrary to strategic needs, seldom change rapidly over time. The historic failure of many firms to adjust to new substitute technologies and develop or adopt them may result more from the rigidity of organizational practices than from technical incompetence.[36] The current difficulties of major pharmaceutical groups in developing and exploiting biotechnologies, compared with genetic engineering start-ups, may result from similar difficulty in adjusting managerial attitudes and organizational processes to new requirements. Known rigidity of internal conditions within a firm may lead a thoughtful top management to over-adjust to strategic needs in anticipation of organizational adaptation lags. Extensive differentiation may thus be sought, even when technologies are quite interdependent, when the demands put on the organization to successfully develop and implement the new required technologies or business concepts would quickly involve major departures from current practice within the organization. For example, IBM reversed several organizational dogmas to adjust to the requirements of an emerging PC business (*e.g.*, relying on outside vendors for key components and assemblies, accepting independent distribution channels, going for an "open architecture"). Yet IBM's PC team simplified its task somewhat by relying on "off-the-shelf" modules and components, calling on known technologies. This minimized the need for technical interdependencies with the rest of IBM. Similarly, the fact that Airbus A300 was state of the art, but did not involve really new technology, may have helped its management team make it independent from its multiple European parents, and build an original "businesslike" culture within the venture. In both cases, technical suboptimization may have taken place as the cost for organizational differentiation, but it led to the ultimate success of the venture.

Comparing biotechnologies with IBM's PC venture and with Airbus raises one more interesting issue. In both the PC and the Airbus cases, external signals were clear, and both efforts followed a series of failures (for IBM to compete successfully at the low end of the market and for the European aerospace industry to capture large civilian markets). Failures within the firm could be ascribed to a lack of differentiation, and the need to increase differentiation thus be made legitimate. In biotechnology, signals are less clear, and there are no precedents. The esoteric and intrinsically uncertain nature of the technologies and the vested interests of key members of the organization may make it difficult for top managers to perceive weak signals early.

Differentiation, therefore, is not achieved early enough, and development lags. External signal confirmation may then become disproportionately important. The optimistic forecast about their own activities by genetic engineering start-ups (in order to raise funding) or the opinions of consultants, stockholders or journalists may do more to prompt a recognition of the differentiation needs of biotechnologies in major European health care companies than the weak internal signals that integration into the existing chemical research facilities is not necessarily effective. In sum, a difficult first step is to recognize the need for differentiation early enough to be useful.

Similarly, the benefits from interdependencies at later stages may go unheeded. The existing businesses may ignore the venture, and the venture management may be more concerned with maintaining autonomy than with corporate overall optimization. In other cases, the interdependencies may become obvious and create strong pressures for integration. For example, IBM's Entry System Division, which developed IBM's PC quite independently (as an independent business unit) came under direct company control and guidance starting in 1983. Not only had the size of the PC business become significant to IBM, but also—and more critically, as the product evolved from stand-alone to part of a network—it had become much more interdependent with other IBM businesses. Microcomputer manufacturers with less of a stake in other segments of the information technology industry could continue to rely on project teams or development units for their new products (*e.g.*, Apple's Mackintosh team) as did companies aimed at the remaining "stand-alone" applications.

As the competitive structure of the industry shifted from small, dedicated firms to divisions of major electronics companies (*e.g.*, DEC, Hewlett-Packard, NEC), the strategic significance of the PC business also shifted—for a company such as IBM—from being independent to becoming critical to a wider range of businesses against common competitors. All these reasons called for great integration of the PC business development effort into other activities in the company. In early 1985, the PC business lost its independent marketing function; this made it very close, in terms of management and organizational interdependencies, to other IBM product lines. Resources (*e.g.*, laboratories and scientists) may not be shared among several programs, and corporate pressures may exist to develop common components or to rely on existing ones. Deciding when to enforce conformity, and to force reliance on corporate capabilities, and when to leave units free to interact, or not, with other units, therefore is an important issue.

Organization Contexts to Manage Innovation and Interdependencies: Toward a Framework

In the previous sections have been described the main capabilities required to manage technological innovation so as to exploit the interdependencies existing in large, complex firms. These capabilities are unlikely to be created and maintained without direct top management involvement. They require active management. We, therefore, turn now to the means available to top management for influencing the capabilities described above.

A Typical Repertory of Administrative Mechanisms

Building on the process school of policy research (for a summary, see Bower and Doz), our prior research work has pointed the way to the importance of richly structured organization contexts to successfully manage ambiguous situations and complex trade-offs.[37] It has led to an analysis and an assessment of tools used by top management to balance international integration and national responsiveness priorities in international operations.[38] An indicative range of mechanisms typically used in large, complex firms in managing trade-offs and achieving balance between responding to the diversity of market conditions and obtaining advantages from their global presence is provided in Table 1.

A similar range of mechanisms as presented in Table 1 may provide leverage points for top management to vary the levels of interdependence and differentiation in the innovation process.

Information systems, for instance, may help or hinder the development of multiple perspectives, according to whether they allow the company to be considered as alternate sets of portfolios, according to the purpose being pursued. Typically, product, application, technology and function-specific perspectives need to be sustained without too much difficulty. While one can argue that *ad hoc* analysis and study can always be done in one perspective or another and be an eye-opener for management, experiences show that—for a perspective to endure and be effectively represented in decision-making—it must somehow be embedded in the routine management process, starting with the accounting, control and information systems.

Information systems must also be clear enough to identify factor risks, and to monitor progress to relate outcomes to causes. A critical issue here is that usual accounting systems are relatively poor at depicting accurately innovation activities where costs are investments, and where their structure and evolution are uncertain. Multiple analytical perspectives also facilitate the development of plural resource allocation channels, and provide the infrastructure for realistic multiple overlapping planning processes (periods, products, projects, and programs). Changes may also be facilitated; a change in differentiation only involves temporarily and locally deactivating certain management tools (*e.g.*, exempting an entrepreneurial venture from the usual requirements of the planning process).

Conversely, increases in interdependence only involve reactivating and emphasizing already existing management tools over time. The process of change is greatly facilitated because the administrative infrastructure is already in place.

Mechanisms are also mutually reinforcing; multiple foci in information systems facilitate flexibility in resource allocation. In turn, the use of multiple resource allocation channels provides credibility to multiple perspectives and shows their need. Similarly, measurement systems facilitate or hinder innovation. They may—by bundling and unbundling activities—allow a better assessment of individual risks and foster clearer commitments, and allow measurement that explains and analyses the causes of good or poor performance, thus making it easier for managers to assume well-delineated risks and to negotiate their own performance evaluation.

TABLE 1. A typical repertoire of administrative mechanisms

I. Data Management Mechanisms	II. Managers' Management Mechanisms	III. Conflict Resolution Mechanisms
1. Information Systems	1. Choice of Key Managers	1. Decision Responsibility Assignments
2. Measurement Systems	2. Career Paths	2. Integrators
3. Resource Allocation Procedures	3. Reward and Punishment Systems	3. Business Terms
4. Strategic Planning	4. Management Development	4. Coordination Committees
5. Budgeting Process	5. Patterns of Socialization	5. Task Forces
		6. Issue Resolution Processes

A complete description of how each tool listed in Table 1 can be structured and used to contribute to the five critical organizational capabilities listed in the previous section would be too long to be detailed here, and too abstract to be useful. It is also at least partly situational, its details varying with the nature of the industry, the underlying technologies, and the involved firm. The relative size, time horizon, number of individual projects, and their complexity put more or less taxing demands on the management systems.

It is also important to acknowledge the intrinsic differences between tools in how flexibly they can be used and how quickly they do—or do not—show results. Task forces may be seen as temporary mechanisms leading to quick results. Major changes in strategic planning procedures may take several years to yield results; shifts in career patterns may take even longer. Some mechanisms may involve high continuity in less visible ways. Views held by individual managers, which support specific resource allocation proposals and discard others, are shaped over a period of time by perceptions of benefits and risks, by the development of careers, and by the building of personal track records. Though the formal approval criteria for projects may be changed easily, as can the format of these proposals, the views that can actually kill a proposal or propel it toward corporate approval cannot be modified rapidly. Managers do not respond immediately—or even quickly—to new mechanisms. Therefore, it is critical for top management to consider carefully the time required for a mechanism to bear results and the delays involved in shifting the focus of a mechanism.

Time horizons of mechanisms are obvious limitations to agility, yet the differences in time horizons can be used constructively. Mechanisms that can be reset most quickly, or from which specific units can be exempted (*e.g.*, the planning system) can be used to increase differentiation and encourage innovation. Mechanisms that cannot be changed rapidly (*e.g.*, how the career patterns are evolving and how they are read by other executives) can be used to provide stability, to limit perceived risks, and to give clear, unchanging rules of the game and its values. Individual managers can also understand a few constant parameters (*e.g.*, stable employment policies with incentives for innovation and internal venture success, but no overnight millionaires), and trust they will remain over time. There may be multiple games (*e.g.*, different measurement, evaluation and reward criteria) according to where in the organization one is located, but the rules for each game must be clear and explicit, and expected not to change suddenly. In sum, some long-term horizon mechanisms may be used to provide invariant "givens" for daily risks and set norms of behavior, while shorter time horizon mechanisms are used to provide variety and to allow the differentiation of innovative efforts.

Two Illustrative Cases

While it is too early in our research program to describe projects in complete detail (and space considerations would prevent it here, anyway) a few comments can be provided to contrast different approaches to organizational context as used in two different projects. Since the data on neither have yet been released by the involved companies, their descriptions will have to remain anonymous and somewhat abstract.

Both companies A and B started technology and product development efforts in technological and competitive domains adjacent to their existing activities. In both cases, these efforts required significant departures from usual practice to succeed. Patterns of resource commitments at various stages in technology and product development, underlying technical bases, potential competitors, and likely critical success factors in the marketplace differed significantly between A's and B's traditional businesses and the new efforts. In both cases, however, it was clear that the new efforts would not be devoid of consequences in terms of technology, manufacturing and competitive dynamics to the existing businesses. Existing businesses also had to contribute technology and expertise to the new ventures. Interdependencies existed, both in terms of sharing core technologies and of reaching common customers.

Company A

Company A set up a separate project with a few scientists and business development experts. After exploring the technical and market feasibility of the technologies and of the business concepts which these could allow, it was decided in principle to set up a separate venture if the initial separate project was successful. The new venture was set aside from the main lines of activities. A venture manager was selected from within upper middle management of business units; he was the first to accept the challenge to run the project and the venture who also had—in the view of top management—the necessary technical and managerial capabilities. The effort was shielded from "interference" from the existing businesses (whose managers had for years maintained that such a project was not practically feasible and had no market, anyway).

Usual planning and budgeting procedures—particularly sophisticated in Company A—were relaxed and not imposed upon the new operation. Its new managers "only" had to make a series of presentations of the new project when it moved from R&D status to new internal venture group status with its own manufacturing, marketing, and sales capabilities and resources. Usual procedures for resource allocation were also simplified, and many of the intermediate reporting levels and corporate checks and balances procedures were removed. The new manager could recruit from within the organization—with the support of top management, who provided a sense of urgency for the transfers to the new venture—and from outside. An informal "board" of top managers was created to oversee the venture, and to assure that other units—which were operating within a rather bureaucratic planning and control system—would be satisfied that "control" was somehow exercised on the new venture.

This very clearly was increasing the differentiation and autonomy of the new effort as it moved from an embryonic research effort to an emerging business.

Difficulties surfaced, however, with managers' management. The bureaucratic nature of the formal organization of Company A was counterbalanced by an informal "clan" culture, which circumvented some of the relative rigidity of the formal systems. When the new venture was created, therefore, its managers remained salaried employees with no direct financial incentive linked to venture results and performance. Initially the enthusiasm for the project and the excitement of running a "whole" business were sufficient to maintain commitment among middle managers who, for the first time, had a complete general management perspective (all the managers of the venture management team were functional specialists, whose prior experience had been in specialized technical jobs in large divisions). After some time, however, particularly as they relied upon outside small subcontractors, who made considerable personal incomes from supplying A's venture, the venture managers started to feel that their efforts were not well rewarded.

Furthermore, as the venture succeeded and grew, some of the original members of the team fell back into specialized jobs within the venture and lost the excitement of being closely associated with its running. General management experience took precedence in promotion decisions within the venture over specialized excellence, adding to the frustration of some of the original members. Dissonance was created in the perceptions of managers between—on the one side—data management and conflict resolution mechanisms, which encouraged strong differentiations and—on the other side—managers' management mechanisms, which still functioned mainly on the premise of "clan" regulated and encouraged integration.

Managers who had tasted autonomy and entrepreneurship felt inadequately rewarded for their efforts, particularly at middle levels within the venture. Some considered leaving. By contrast, top management of the venture felt rewarded in (1) the opportunity to run a separate business at a relatively early age; (2) the expectation of running another such operation in the future; and (3) the hope that their careers would move faster as a result of the experience and visibility obtained from running the venture. They would accommodate the dissonance between how their business was related to the company (via market mechanisms) and how they—as individuals—related to the company (via clan mechanisms).

A little later, once the venture began to look like a success, it was transformed into a regular corporate division, and relationships with the other divisions were strongly encouraged by top management (who gradually withdrew the shield they had put over the venture). This partial reinsertion was felt as painful and difficult by the venture's managers, who were concerned that their innovativeness and entrepreneurship might be stifled.

Yet Company A had succeeded in varying interdependencies and differentiation over time with a good measure of success, successfully developing a new innovative business where prior attempts had met with skepticism and never taken off. Despite some of the tensions created among middle-level executives, it also succeeded in retaining all key personnel through two difficult transitions—from integration to autonomy and differentiation, and back again.

Company B

Company B, faced with a potential innovation raising similar issues, approached the situation quite differently. It decided to set up a separate research center in a distinct physical location, to regroup its own experts there, and to hire individual scientists from outside the company. The concept was to create a self-contained effort as in Company A and to shield it from pressures. Top management support, however, was not translated into specific alterations to existing management mechanisms. The decision to build a new research center was slow, as were the approvals for hiring young top-notch scientists who did not easily fall within the existing (low) salary scales of a big bureaucratic company.

Further, even though the innovation required a more intimate cooperation among R&D, process engineering, marketing, and business planning functions (as a new venture would provide), the effort remained largely contained within the R&D group. No such thing as an independent venture was created. Research managers found that it was difficult to differentiate their efforts and to acquire and use the necessary human resources, since the research hierarchy remained controlled by senior managers who sometimes lacked an understanding of—and sympathy toward—the new technologies.

In a fast-moving field, internal resource allocation choices remained a slow process, while cooperative agreements with external parties usually bogged down in innumerable negotiation and discussion sessions. As the scientists retained a narrow focus, they missed the opportunity to present to top management a wider view from which they could more easily have earned support.

Vertical functional hierarchies prevented marketing or business development experts from exercising a significant influence on the choice of new research programs within the unit. Similarly, manufacturability considerations came almost as an afterthought. Since, in the new business—more so than in Company B's traditional activities, which were well known by management—analyses of application choices, market focus, and scale-up problems were critical to R&D choices, and these inputs were not provided, Company B went down several dead-ends in moving toward product development. Within the new research groups, researchers remained preoccupied mainly with their own pet scientific projects, rather than with the development of a coherent research team.

The usual regulation mode of the existing activities, where R&D was institutionalized as a routine activity, was carried over into the new activity with little recognition of the need for differentiation. Integration was not performed, either, since the new field could not rely on the bureaucratic procedures of the older fields. As a result, Company B soon lagged behind other companies in innovation in this particular technology and market.

Recognition of the Need for Differentiations

Why did Company B fail where Company A succeeded? Most of the difficulties came from senior management levels not recognizing the need for differentiations. Part of the issue came from the unicity of perspective within the organization, where technical problems are solved by giving additional resources to R&D, not by differentiating their use. The R&D establishments, used to working with great independence, did not accept easily that business development managers have a greater say, and that interfaces with manufacturing and production should be more intense. The problems and opportunities were never brought up to top management in a comprehensive way. Faced with fragmented evidence, top management was slow to react to issues and problems and to perceive opportunity. Despite the initial investment in a new center, the project fell into the resource allocation trap described earlier: Aware of the technical uncertainties, research managers asked for incremental resources, and were slow in deploying them. Even for those who saw the need to do things differently, the perceived risks were too high, and they did not voice their concerns loudly enough nor take drastic action.

Several tentative implications (or further research questions or hypotheses) can be drawn from this somewhat casual analysis:

- To achieve both differentiation and integration in the management of innovations that have strong interdependencies — actual or potential — with existing activities involves the use of a series of administrative mechanisms, some focused on the management of data, others on the management of individuals and groups, and still others on the management of conflicts and tensions.

- In the development of a typical innovation, changing priorities between integration and differentiation can be implemented via selective alterations to administrative mechanisms. Understanding the use of mechanisms, their potential to encourage differentiation and integration, according to how they are set, is important. Mechanisms also differ in their time horizons for both resetting them and for their impact to be felt. Differences in time horizon can be used selectively to provide for both continuity and variety.

- Not changing the setting of mechanisms makes differentiation and change extremely difficult (as in our Company B example), while changing all mechanisms may create much uncertainty and confusion and excessively weaken the existing culture without providing any consistent alternative. The company may emerge much weakened from overall change. Since corporate culture is, by and large, the cumulative effect over time of a set of mechanisms used with continuity, it is important that some mechanisms be invariant, while others change. Some dissonance is needed between various mechanisms, but such dissonance must be kept within bounds. Various managers in various positions within the organization may tolerate dissonance more or less easily.

- Human beings adjust and respond to new mechanisms or to newly reset mechanisms with varying speeds. Speed depends partly on corporate culture (*e.g.*, managers at General Electric respond very fast to changes in the administrative mechanisms, while managers in companies with strong "family" traditions may be less easily influenced.) National cultures may also play a role (*e.g.*, the US vs. The Netherlands vs. Japan). Fast resetting of mechanisms to best match differentiation and integration needs in rapidly evolving fields with short product life-cycles and strong pressures for reducing development time may be ineffective. Individual human response time may be a pacing factor in shifting differentiation and integration between innovative and operational activities.

- At a given point in time, different regulating modes among managers may coexist in various parts of the company. The internal management team of a new venture may well function as a clan, but be related to other parts of the corporation by market mechanisms; or research labs may be a hierarchy, but connected via network mechanisms to the users of their research. This implies the existence of boundary-spanning roles (*e.g.*, West's role in Kidder's account of the development of a new computer at Data General) in various positions in the company. Managers in these roles have to function simultaneously within several regulating modes, according to the relationships they are involved in. This is conceptually different from gatekeeper's roles,[39] since it involves not only the circulation of information, but a wide range of behaviors and a more direct activity in decision-making. Some of the roles traditionally defined as "champion," "sponsor," "internal entrepreneur," etc., can be interpreted in boundary-spanning terms.

● These issues of boundary-spanning capabilities between units working according to different modes of regulation are magnified in cooperative agreements particularly between large and small firms. Typically, the large firm will cooperate with the small one because the small one has some unique technology to offer. Within the small firm the relationship with the big one is usually handled from the very top, and with an "arm's-length" attitude which stems both from the concern of being taken over (or just imbricated into the large firm) and from the fact that entrepreneurs heading small firms have more affinity and familiarity with market mechanisms than with hierarchies, clans or networks. Within the large firm, however, the relationship will usually be handled by middle-level research executives, who attempt to practice clan, network or hierarchy approaches, either to better embrace the small firm (and ensure the full transfer of its technology) or by habit because it is the usual mode in which they function within the large firm. Such conflicts in regulating modes may limit the results of cooperative agreements— and their value to both parties. Unless they are recognized and explicitly managed, they may also create tremendous misunderstandings, and result in the premature dissolution of cooperative agreements.

Conclusion

In this article, we have set an agenda for top management to facilitate the success of innovations in the context of large, complex companies. While autonomous entrepreneurial ventures are useful, they are not the panacea that popular management literature sometimes likens them to. Our focus has been on what both autonomous entrepreneurial ventures and divisional R&D efforts neglect or severely suboptimize, namely, core or system technologies with strong interdependencies with existing businesses and technologies.

In our view, the task includes maintaining multiple perspectives on the total portfolio of corporate activities for environmental scanning and planning purposes; providing flexible resource allocation channels to allow corporate, business unit, and individual innovation and entrepreneurship; managing personal risks and rewards explicitly; mixing various approaches to the management of people (hierarchy, market, clan, network); and providing flexibility in shifting the balance between differentiation and interdependence in the development of an innovation over time. The above agenda requires active management. Without direct top management action, the above conditions are unlikely to endure in a large, complex firm. In the last section we proposed an approach toward creating the conditions summarized above.

Notes

1. Raymond Vernon, "The Product Life Hypothesis in a New Environment," *Oxford Bulletin of Economics and Statistics* 41:4 (November 1979), pp. 255–267. See also Gary Hamel and C.K. Prahalad, "Creating Global Strategic Capability" in Dan Schendel, Neil Hood and Jan-Erik Vahlne, eds., *Strategies in Global Competition* (London: John Wiley, forthcoming, 1986).
2. Rosabeth Moss Kanter, *The Change Masters* (New York: Simon & Schuster, 1983).
3. Michel Crozier, *The Bureaucratic Phenomenon* (Chicago: University of Chicago Press, 1967).
4. Joseph L. Bower, *Managing the Resource Allocation Process* (Boston: Harvard Business School Division of Research, 1970).
5. See Howard Stevenson and David E. Gumpert, "The Heart of Entrepreneurship," *Harvard Business Review*, March–April 1985, pp. 85–94; and Andrew van de Ven and Andre L. Delbecq, "Determinants of Coordination Modes Within Organisations," *American Sociology Review* 41 (April 1976), pp. 322–338.
6. See James Brian Quinn, "Technological Innovation, Entrepreneurship and Strategy," *Sloan Management Review* 20:3 (1979), pp. 19–30; see also James Brian Quinn, "Managing Innovation: Controlled Chaos," *Harvard Business Review*, May–June 1985, pp. 73–84; Norman D. Fast, "The Future of Industrial New Venture Departments," *Industrial Marketing Management* 8 (1979), pp. 264–279; and Thomas J. Peters and Robert H. Waterman, Jr., *In Search of Excellence* (New York: Harper & Row, 1982).
7. Norman D. Fast, "The Future of Industrial New Venture Departments," *op. cit.*
8. Robert A. Burgelman, "A Process Model of Internal Corporate Venturing in the Diversified Major Firm," *Administrative Science Quarterly* 28 (1983), pp. 223–244.
9. See R.M. Adams, "An Approach to New Business Ventures," *Research Management* 12 (1969), pp. 255–260; and R.T. Wallace, "New Venture Management at Owens Illinois," *Research Management* 12 (1969), pp. 261–270.
10. See *Business Week*, April 18, 1983, pp. 52–54; and *Industry Week*, August 20, 1984, pp. 39–48.
11. Norman D. Fast, "The Future of Industrial New Venture Departments," *op. cit.*; and Robert A. Burgelman, "Managing the New Venture Division: Research Findings and Implications for Strategic Management," *Strategic Management Journal* 6 (1985).
12. Marjorie A. Lyles (research in progress).
13. Robert A. Burgelman, "Designs for Corporate Entrepreneurs in Established Firms," *California Management Review* 6:3 (Spring 1984), pp. 154–166.
14. Gary Hamel and C.K. Prahalad, "Creating Global Strategic Capability," in Schendel *et al.*, *op. cit.*
15. See Euroconsult, "Le Bonzai de l'Industrie Japonaise," *Bulletin CPE*, no. 40 (July 1984).
16. A joint INSEAD-University of Michigan project is underway to analyze the management of innovation in large, complex firms with the support of such companies as Ciba Geigy, Philips, Elf Aquitaine, General Electric, GTE and others. The principal investigators are Professors Doz and Angelmar at INSEAD, and Professor Prahalad at the University of Michigan. Parallel research is being undertaken in Japan by Professors Nonaka, Sakakibara and Takeuchi (Hitotsubashi University); Kogono (Kobe University); and Okumura (Keio University) to pursue such investments.
17. See Balaji S. Chakravarthy, "Strategic Self Renewal: A Planning Framework for Today," *Academy of Management Review* 9:3 (1984), pp. 1–12.
18. For a description, see Nippon Electric Co. Ltd., HBS Case Services, Harvard Business School, Boston, MA, HBSCS no. 0-383-098 (1982).
19. Raymond Snoddy and Christopher Lorenz, "How Matsushita Averted an Impending Crisis," *Financial Times*, June 14, 1985, p. 28.
20. Robert A. Burgelman, "Designs for Corporate Entrepreneurship in Established Firms," *op. cit.*
21. Jules Schwartz, "The Decision to Innovate," unpublished doctoral dissertation, Harvard Business School, 1973.
22. Tracy Kidder, *The Soul of a New Machine* (Boston: Little Brown, 1981).
23. Modesto Maidique, "Entrepreneurs, Champions and Technological Innovation," *Sloan Management Review* 21:2 (Winter 1980), pp. 59–76.
24. Richard Hamermesh, "The Administration of Strategy," chapter 6, book manuscript, publication forthcoming.
25. See Herbert H. Simon, *Administrative Behavior* (New York: The Free Press, 1945); and Michel Crozier, *The Bureaucratic Phenomenon*, *op. cit.*

26. See William G. Ouchi, "Markets, Bureaucracies and Clans," *Administrative Science Quarterly* (March 1980); also see Rodney Clark, "Aspects of Japanese Commercial Innovation," Technical Change Center Working Paper no. TCCR-84-010.

27. C.K. Prahalad and Yves Doz, *The Work of Top Management* (New York: The Free Press, forthcoming, 1986).

28. Rosabeth Moss Kanter, *The Change Masters, op. cit.*

29. Thomas Peters and Robert H. Waterman, Jr., *In Search of Excellence, op. cit.*

30. Mariann Jelinek, *Institutionalizing Innovation: A Study of Organizational Learning Systems* (New York: Praeger, 1979).

31. M. Moritz, *The Little Kingdom: The Private Story of Apple Computer* (Morrow, 1984); "Apple Computer's Counterattack Against IBM," *Business Week*, January 16, 1984; "Apple Bites Back," *Fortune*, February 20, 1984.

32. Thomas Lifson, "The Sogo Shosha: Strategy, Structure and Culture," unpublished dissertation, Department of Sociology, Harvard University, 1978; Anders Edstrom and Jay Galbraith, "Transfer of Managers As a Co-ordination and Control Strategy," *Administrative Science Quarterly* 22 (1977), pp. 248–263.

33. See Thomas A. Allen, *Managing the Flow of Technology: Technology Transfer and the Dissemination of Technological Information Within the R&D Organization* (Cambridge, MA: MIT Press, 1977).

34. Thomas Lifson, "The Sogo Shosha: Strategy, Structure and Culture," *op. cit.*

35. See Paul R. Lawrence and G. Dyer, *Renewing American Industry* (New York: The Free Press, 1983).

36. Arnold C. Cooper and Dan Schendel, "Strategic Responses to Technological Threats," *Business Horizons* 19 (1976), pp. 61–69.

37. For a summary analysis of the process school of policy research, see Joseph L. Bower and Yves L. Doz, "Strategy Formulation: A Social and Political Process," in Dan Schendel and Charles W. Hofer, *Strategic Management* (Boston: Little Brown, 1979).

38. See Yves L. Doz, *Multinational Strategic Management* (Oxford: Pergamon Press, 1985); and Yves L. Doz and C.K. Prahalad, "Patterns of Strategic Control Within MNCs," *Journal of International Business Studies*, 15:2 (Fall 1984), pp. 55–72.

39. Thomas A. Allen, *Managing the Flow of Technology.*

Timing Technological Transitions

Richard N. Foster

ABSTRACT. Technological discontinuities are among the most disruptive challenges facing corporations, and they are on the increase. Empirically, it appears that few corporations are able to survive discontinuities. They either lose market share, money or their independence. Despite the importance of the discontinuity problem for top management, few have done much to better anticipate and deal with these increasingly frequent events. They act as if they assume that there is nothing that can be done. The problem appears to be one of misplaced faith in some conventional assumptions about what it takes to succeed. The author examines these assumptions, particularly those dealing with the supposed advantages of defenders, and pinpoints their errors. This knowledge then leads to positive solutions that hopefully, in turn, will lead to increased success for some of our most important companies.

When the transistor replaced the vacuum tube in the mid-1950s, every one of the top ten producers of vacuum-tube components was caught flat-footed. Six of them discounted the importance of the new development and held aloof from solid-state technology, while the other four tried to change horses, but failed. Not one of the ten is a force in today's $10 billion semiconductor industry.

This familiar scenario is not confined to high-technology industries. Consider tire cords. Sixty years ago they were made of cotton. Then — in the mid-1940s — the lead shifted to rayon and the American Viscose Company became the leading supplier of cord. Early in the 1960s, however, Du Pont's nylon tire cords captured the top position. The lead shifted yet again in the late 1970s, when Celanese took control with its polyester fibers. Each time a new technology superseded the old, industry leadership changed hands.

Few companies, it seems, are able to make a successful transition to a profitable new technology. Typically, technology leaders wake up too late to the threat of a new technology.

How do technologies mature? Why is the process so often accompanied by management paralysis and competitive dislocation? And what steps can companies take to improve their ability to anticipate and manage transitions between technologies, reducing the chances of such dislocation in the face of future technological change? These are the questions that will be explored here.

Richard N. Foster is a Director of McKinsey & Company and heads the firm's Technology practice. He is the author of a book on successfully managing through technological discontinuities, which will be published in early 1986.

Technological Limits and Potential

Technological improvement in any field is ultimately limited by the laws of nature. The number of transistors that can be placed on a silicon chip is limited by the crystal structure of silicon, the ultimate strength of a fiber by the strength of its intermolecular bonds.

Most industries are far from these ultimate natural barriers, and much more likely to come up against practical technological limits. The efficiency of today's car engines, for instance, is limited by the ability of existing engine alloys to withstand heat; hence, researchers are investigating the possibility of using ceramics in their place.

The mission of research and development is to advance toward the limit—both practical and theoretical—of a particular technology. How much improvement is possible is determined by the difference between the current state of the art and the technical limit. This difference can be called the *technical potential*. As the state of the art nears its technical limits, each increment of research effort produces less improvement since the most effective ideas presumably have already been used. Said another way, as the limits of technology are approached, the returns from further R&D diminish. Many companies don't understand where the limits of their technologies lie, and finding out can be a complicated business. But the payoff can be great.

In the late 1960s, for example, IBM investigated the limits of computer technology.[1] Thorough evaluation at the Watson Research Labs confirmed the prevalent assumption that these limits were ultimately set by the accuracy with which computer circuits could be printed by photolithography. It also disclosed, however, that the state of the art of component design, device design, and—most particularly—chip "package" design all posed more restrictive practical limits. To get around these limits, the scientists changed the existing design in what became known as the "multiple stacked array" concept on which IBM's 4300 Series computers were based—a major market success of the 1970s that would have been impossible without thorough understanding of technological limits.

The role of technology in corporate strategy is directly related to technological potential. If the potential is high—*i.e.*, if the state of the art is remote from the technical limit (a situation typical of "high-tech" industries)—technology is likely to be an important element in the strategy of the business. If the technological potential is low, then other business functions are likely to loom larger.

The S-Curve Phenomenon

Of necessity, all R&D work is carried out in the context of technical limits. Early in an R&D program, knowledge bases need to be built, lines of inquiry must be drawn and tested, and technical problems surfaced. Researchers need to investigate and discard unworkable approaches. Thus, until this knowledge has been acquired, the pace of progress toward technological limits is usually slow. But then it picks up, typically reaching a maximum when something like half the technical potential has been realized. At this point, the technology begins to be constrained by its lim-

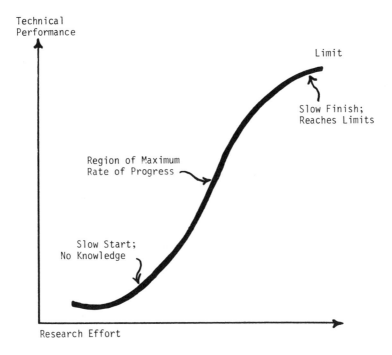

FIGURE 1. The S-curve phenomenon.

its, and the rate of performance improvement begins to slow. Diminishing returns set in. This phenomenon can be depicted as an S-curve. Figure 1 shows the concept schematically, while Figure 2 displays a representative set of actual S-curves from the tire cord industry.

In the case of the tire cords for bias-ply passenger tires, technical performance is defined in terms of the combined parameters used by the B.F. Goodrich Company in evaluating suppliers' offerings. These include tensile strength, abrasion and corrosion resistance, and adhesion to the rubber carcass of the tire — all factors related to desired end-product attributes, such as dimensional stability, longevity and cost. The cumulative R&D effort usually can be measured in man-years of R&D effort, or, as it is in this example, in dollars of R&D investment.

What is important to remember is that, no matter how vigorously a competitor backs its own technology, it cannot escape the realities of technical limits and the implications of the S-curve. Inevitably, the technology with the greatest potential takes control of the market. At the same time, competitive leadership is all too likely to change hands.

R&D productivity, like manufacturing productivity, may be defined as the ratio of the change in output to the change in input — *i.e.*, the improvement in the performance of the product or process divided by the incremental effort required. Accordingly, R&D productivity is determined by the relationship between technical progress and R&D investment at various stages of development. For example, Du Pont, pursuing a later stage advance in nylon, was getting 0.08 units of progress per $1 million of R&D investment. Its competitor, Celanese, then in the midstage

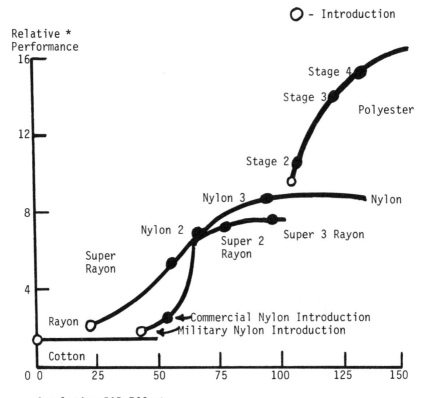

*An index used by tire cord customers to evaluate tire cord
performance when compared to the performance of cotton,
which has a performance rating of 1.0.

**FIGURE 2. S-curves in tire cord technology
Source: McKinsey analysis.**

of polyester development, was getting 0.33 units of improvement per $1 million of effort, four times as much as Du Pont.[2] Also, polyester tire cord was already superior to nylon, so Celanese was making faster progress on a better product. No company can withstand such competition for long. As Celanese's victory over the redoubtable Du Pont demonstrated, in technological contests the attacker often has a decisive economic advantage.

Sometimes, of course, market factors can actually cancel the day of reckoning. The end objective, after all, is not R&D productivity, but R&D return: the profit earned on the R&D investment. R&D productivity is only one of the two variables determining R&D return; the other is the profit made from a given technical advance. This variable, which can be called the *R&D yield*, is a function of the competitive structure of the industry: supply/demand conditions, relative power of customers and suppliers, company strategies, substitute products, external influences, and so on.

Decisions about which technology to work on and when to invest in it should be made on the basis of returns, and should involve both productivity and yield. Examining returns in terms of technological progress (productivity) and the economic value of that progress (yield) has organizational advantages, too. R&D productivity is determined largely by the R&D strategy and the efficiency of the R&D department in pursuing that strategy. Thus, controlling and improving R&D productivity is largely within the power of the R&D department. Yield, on the other hand, is the result of market conditions and competitor strategies, subjects that are the traditional responsibilities of the business units. R&D productivity and yield ultimately need to be coupled, of course, but this is best done after they have been examined independently.

Breaking down returns into productivity and yield also provides a more precise sense of the sources of low returns. For returns to be high, both productivity and yield need to be substantial. If either is low, their product will be low. If productivity is high and yield is low or negative, as it might be if there is a prospect for continued overcapacity in the industry, then returns will be low or negative. Accordingly, projects in this area should not be pursued, despite substantial technical potential and high productivity. Nor do projects make sense where yield is substantial, but the technology is mature. The low productivity of the mature technology indicates that little technical progress can be made. Investments in manufacturing, logistics, or marketing might be more productive. Companies that manage their technology well have recognized these pitfalls, and learned to avoid them.

The Impact of Discontinuities

By focusing R&D on improving the performance of current technology, companies limit themselves to evolutionary progress along a single S-curve until rapidly diminishing returns signal the imminent approach of technical limits. In failing to investigate the potential of new technologies, they often miss opportunities to exploit powerful competitive leverage.

Such opportunities, however, are not always easy to grasp. Almost by definition, the S-curves of different technologies are not linked. The gaps that separate them are often both substantial and strategically important, and to manage the transition is a difficult and delicate task.

The tire and cord technologies discussed previously, for example, are linked to bias-ply tires—a construction technology that has its own S-curve and its own technological potential, which happens to be significantly less than that of the newer radial construction. Goodyear clung to its bias-ply construction, which was beaten out by the Michelin-backed radials, just as Du Pont, sticking to nylon, was bested by Celanese. It is easier to detect a technological discontinuity from afar than it is when you are right in the middle of one.

One reason why it is so difficult to detect a technological discontinuity from the inside is that an existing competitor has more to lose with the introduction of a new technology, while a new entrant has little to lose and a great deal to gain. In tire cords, Du Pont felt it needed to protect its existing nylon plant assets. Celanese had no such need; it only felt a need to utilize its new polyester facilities. The need to protect its assets may have helped Du Pont believe that polyester had little market potential. History shows that this was wishful thinking.

This blindness to the advantages of new technology has affected almost all industries at one time or another. In electronics, the dramatic discontinuity seen in the shift from vacuum tubes to transistors was followed by a succession of further discontinuities as transistors gave way to SSI, to LSI, and then to microprocessors. In metal packaging, the move from three-piece to two-piece cans represents an important discontinuity (the retort pouch may be another). In each case, a technological discontinuity led to a competitive dislocation—and technology leaders became losers.

The essence of managing technology well, it seems, is the ability to make smooth and timely transitions to new technologies with superior performance improvement potential—in other words, to cross discontinuities effectively. In many cases, this ability may be the only key to the problems of declining R&D productivity and deteriorating competitive position. Superior operational efficiency in R&D can rarely, if ever, compensate for an inferior technical strategy.

Technological Myopia

Strategic errors, however, are not always to blame when a technology leader is overtaken by a competitor. Incorrect perceptions of technical limits, inability to measure technological progress, faulty interpretation of market signals, and unrealistic faith in "understanding customer needs" tend to mask the deterioration that sets in when an existing technology matures and the superior potential of an alternative begins to affect the competitive balance.

Managements unaccustomed to thinking in terms of technological limits and systematically measuring changes in technical performance almost always grossly overestimate the improvement potential of existing technology. It is tempting to assume that the rapid progress that occurs midway through the S-curve will continue and, unless technical performance *per se* is carefully monitored, the gap between reality and expectation is typically perceived too late—on a 10- or 20-year S-curve, perhaps five to seven years too late.

Knowing when to investigate new technologies is certainly important. On a symmetrical S-curve, half the potential for improving the technology typically remains to be exploited when R&D productivity has reached its maximum. At the midpoint, the bugs are out of the system, cash flow has turned positive, and the business has begun to make a decent profit. It may seem economically perverse to begin investing in a new technology when there is still a lot of potential left in the old. But since it can easily take five or 10 years to develop a new technology, this is often the best time to begin the move by shifting the focus of R&D.

Managers intent on lowering break-even points and improving profits are normally inclined to build bigger plants and spread their overhead over more products. They segment markets to squeeze maximum profit out of customer groups. They work to reduce fixed and overhead costs. All these measures help to maximize profits. And increasing profits tend, in turn, to justify further investment—especially when decisions are based on accounting and financial criteria alone. Only when aggregate financial measures have been broken down into their components, is it possible to distinguish between technological progress and economic returns, and gain real insight into the underlying forces at work.

While R&D concentrates on extracting marginal improvements from old technology, windows of opportunity open up for competitors. And, when a competitor does move in with a new technology, the company's response is typically to increase its investment in the old. But, in choosing to defend an existing technology, rather than displace it with a new one, management only increases the inherent economic advantage of the attacker by enabling him to develop his product or process unhampered by entrenched competitors.

When the first steamships were launched in the mid-19th century, established sailing-ship builders set about improving their design technology, and were building vessels that carried more sail, had faster hulls, and required smaller crews. But the result was only a brief reprieve for a mature technology, not an escape from the S-curve. Thanks to the far greater technological potential of steamships, sails eventually disappeared from the world's shipping lanes.

Sylvania, for another example, was hamstrung by this sailing-ship phenomenon when transistors made their commercial debut. Despite announced plans to move into solid-state technology, it kept on pouring R&D effort into increasingly sophisticated vacuum-tube designs, bringing out complex multi-functional units as late as 1968. Some evidence suggests that, despite Sylvania's public comments to the contrary, the company still believed that the vacuum-tube had a future. For example, Sylvania was an active member of the Electron Tube Information Committee, which was established to explain the advantages of vacuum-tubes and the disadvantages of solid-state devices to the public. In its efforts to wrest incremental performance improvement from its outmoded vacuum-tube technology, Sylvania got aboard the solid-state S-curve too late with too little effort to become a force in the new market.

Misreading Market Signals

The tendency to discount signs of market penetration by new competitors is another costly common error. New products are typically introduced in market niches where they can be highly competitive — niches apparently too small or insufficiently related to the core market to provoke an immediate competitive reaction from the industry leader. Yet, even in a growing market, when the defending producer's sales begin to level off, management often misreads this as a sign of predictable market maturation. And, as the substitution process gathers momentum, the company's sales actually begin to sag. Finally, as the challenger penetrates deeply into its heartland markets, sales collapse and profits swiftly deteriorate — almost before the defender realizes that the battle has begun. It is already too late.

Consider the pattern of substitution cases already mentioned. Polyester tire cords went from a 20 to an 80% share of the bias-ply tire market in 10 years. Radials repeated that market performance against bias-ply tires in four years, and steel tire cords took three years to go from 20 to 80% of the radial tire market. And, in electronics, transistors took seven years to displace vacuum tubes. In each case competitive leadership changed hands.

Part of the problem of recognizing a technological discontinuity is the problem of correctly defining the market. The more mature the product, the more narrowly the market tends to be defined. In the mid-1960s, all tires were bias-ply tires. Hence, by definition, tire-cord makers measured their market performance in terms of their share of the bias-ply tire market. When radial tires entered, the leading tire cord manufacturers should have redefined the market to include tires of any kind, rather than dismissing the radials as "niche fillers." Too many businessmen fail to recognize that any new product—and particularly one based on new technology—potentially redefines the served market.

A final strategic pitfall in technology management is management's tendency to wait for market research cues before committing funds to a new technology. There are three dangers in this perversion of the marketing concept. First, customers are rarely the best judges of potential utility of products that might require them to do things differently; change is painful. Second, the same market cues are available to all qualified suppliers, and the customer, once given the whip hand, can often play suppliers off against one another to advantage, as Boeing has learned to do in the aerospace industry with its materials suppliers. Third, sustained competitive success demands the ability to meet a market need in a unique way. In many businesses it is easy to copy a competitor's market research, but far less easy to copy its technology and harder still to copy its methods of developing new technology. Thus, a company is far more likely to win a real competitive edge by superior technological prowess if the technical potential exists than through any unique knowledge of market needs.

The Culture Trap

The most serious and most elusive impediments to effective technology management, however, are the fundamental cultural weaknesses that underlie the strategic errors being discussed.

A company's product and production technology is an integral part of its corporate culture. Technology directs and conditions management's intuitive strategic responses to opportunities ("can we make a profit on this?"). It conditions the assumptions on which the strategy of the business is based. When the technology changes, the whole corporate culture frequently must change as well. And this is a difficult and painful process.

For electrical engineers designing vacuum tubes in the mid-1950s, the transition to solid-state technology was a real culture shock. To design solid-state devices, they needed to learn an entirely new technical discipline involving a different mathematics. Expert vacuum-tube designers don't necessarily become good solid-state designers. But, because there were enough similarities between the two fields, some vacuum-tube producers assumed that making the transition would not be particularly difficult.

Sometimes a cultural preference for established technology is explicitly built into the management system; several major corporations still give top R&D priority to the defense of their existing product lines. The more doggedly they champion a policy of unyielding technological defense, the more vulnerable to new technology they become. Many R&D vice presidents, having earned their titles by successfully guiding their companies into new technologies, are not disposed to abandon their favorites easily. Indeed, they often inadvertently block the investigation of new and threatening technologies in the name of defending existing product lines.

Traditionally different industries have met technological challenges in different ways. Some observers see the emerging biochemical industry as a wave of the future. If they are correct, how well could established chemical manufacturers cope with the new technological environment? Consider just a few of the differences.

- The chemical business operates large plants whose capacities range from 100 million to one billion pounds a year. Biochemical plants might be small, with typical annual capacities of perhaps from one million to 100 million pounds.
- Whereas chemical plants usually produce a single product, biochemical products could be produced in multiproduct facilities.
- Chemical processes are typically high-temperature operations. Biochemical processes will probably take place at low temperatures, where the energy minimization experience of the chemical industry becomes much less relevant. Biochemical processes will require far tighter processes controls and heavier instrumentation than most chemical processes; thus capital requirements may well differ.
- Biological sterility, generally unnecessary in the chemical industry, is an important requirement in some biochemical processes.

Clearly, to capitalize on the opportunities in biochemicals, established chemical companies would have to do many things differently. As centralized operations become decentralized, strategies, as well as organizational structures, might need to be altered. Management systems might require revision with more authority given to people close to the market and the competition. With shrinking plant size, the role of the plant manager would diminish. New skills and staff needs would develop. New employees, coming from different colleges, universities and disciplines, would move in different cultural circles, and might even speak a different social language. All this would lead to changes in culture, shared values, and management style. The company emerging from such a metamorphosis might resemble its former self in little but name. This transition might be closer than some think. Presently about $1 billion is being spent on biotechnology R&D with perhaps 20% of this going to chemical applications. If the productivity of this work is five to ten times that of conventional chemical R&D, not an uncommon ratio in other transitions, then the total technical programs expected from biochemical research could be on a par with the technical programs expected from all other chemical research.

Cultural barriers to successful technological transitions are particularly difficult to overcome because they are qualitative rather than quantitative. Many managers are accustomed to dealing with strategic issues by creating new research programs or developing new measurement systems; few have experience in changing the entire nature of their companies. But nothing less than that may be called for.

Detecting Decay

Rather than wait passively for a competitive threat to develop, it is necessary for far-sighted management to head off technological decay by addressing the strategic and cultural issues as quickly as they can be detected and identified. A good way to begin is to assess the company's proximity to its technical limits. Typically, certain tell-tale symptoms tend to signal the onset of technological decay:

- *A feeling among top managers that the company's R&D productivity is declining.* Managements that don't measure technological progress have to rely on "gut feel" to know when the S-curve has flattened out. Unfortunately, by the time the flattening can be felt, the game may be lost.

- *A trend toward missed R&D deadlines.* Often interpreted as a sign that the R&D department is losing effectiveness, this may mean that the technology is approaching its limits, thus making performance improvement more difficult to achieve.

- *A shift in the company or industry from product- to process-oriented R&D.* As a technology approaches its limits, process improvements typically replace product improvements as the chief source of technological innovation. Many of our so-called "smokestack" industries are in this situation now. Paradoxically, the best corrective action is a move into unfamiliar product technologies or markets, a risky proposition at best.

- *An apparent loss of productivity in the R&D department.* There is no room for creativity in a technology that is bumping up against its limits.

- *Dissension among the R&D staff.* A particularly frustrating assignment—for example, closing a small gap between the "state of the art" and the technological limit—may turn scientists into pessimists. If the mood of the R&D people is bad, the limits of the technology are probably close.

- *A shift in the sources of sales growth toward narrower market segments.* As we have seen, the final stages of a typical substitution pattern are often dominated by product-line proliferation to meet the needs of small market segments. While this is usually a mandatory economic strategy, it does indicate increasing maturity, and should, therefore, be taken as a signal to look for new "S-curves" that could supersede the present technology.

- *A tendency for significant variations among competitors in R&D spending to produce ever less significant results.* When there is no market advantage to spending more, nor a market disadvantage to spending less, the technology has virtually reached its limits.

- *Dissatisfaction with the performance of a "new broom" R&D manager.* Sometimes a chief executive, frustrated at his company's declining R&D performance, will replace the senior executive with a new, more vibrant R&D manager who is expected to shake the department up and get it going again. He will fail too, if the technology is close to its limits.

- *A trend among smaller, weaker competitors in the industry to invest R&D effort in radical new approaches.* A small company, particularly if it is financially hard pressed, is more likely than an entrenched and profitable producer to invest in a really innovative solution to a customer's problem.

Toward Effective Action

Using these criteria to form an impressionistic assessment of the company's technological health can be an effective prelude to a thorough R&D audit. The audit itself should be based on the principle that R&D effort and R&D investment in a given technology should be proportional to potential for productivity and yield improvement. This principle allows the definition appropriate for R&D strategies (in terms of, say, aggressiveness, risk profile, time for commercial introduction, or a balance of work between old and new markets) to be used in a consistent way for each product line (Figures 3 and 4). These are then compared with actions being taken, or implicit strategies, and the inconsistencies identified. These become the agenda for reshaping the company's R&D program.

Audits of this kind are particularly useful to CEOs of companies with many product lines, since it is typically quite difficult to remember the details of hundreds or thousands of R&D projects. Accurate summaries based on these principles can be extremely useful tools.

These audits frequently reveal that companies are overinvesting in mature technologies and underinvesting in newer ones. In terms of the matrix in Figure 3, this means that companies putting too much emphasis on product lines warranting only "limited defensive support" are not putting enough effort into "heavy emphasis" product lines. To avoid this trap, companies generally will have to take action in two areas in addition to resource reallocations: (1) knowledge building, and (2) measurement and planning systems.

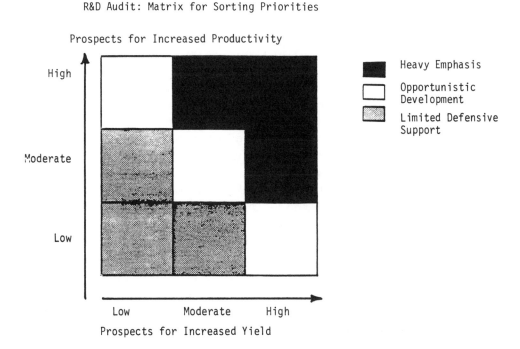

R&D Audit: Matrix for Sorting Priorities

Prospects for Increased Productivity

Heavy Emphasis

Opportunistic Development

Limited Defensive Support

Prospects for Increased Yield

FIGURE 3. R&D Audit: Matrix for Sorting Priorities

	Heavy Emphasis	Opportunistic Development	Limited/Defensive Support
Appropriate Funding	High	Moderate	Low
Expected Payoff	Long-term	Medium-term	Short-term
Acceptable Technical Task	High	Moderate	Low
Primary Focus of Work	Balance New & Existing	Existing Products	Existing Processes
Appropriate Level of Basic Research	High	Low	Very Low

FIGURE 4. R&D Audit: Typical Strategic Implications

Knowledge building. Since a major source of mistakes in technology resource allocation is inadequate knowledge about the limits of present and potential future technologies, efforts to correct this problem are obviously in order, but the utility of knowledge does not stop there. The new knowledge can also be useful in controlling the costs of development. A Rand Corporation study,[3] conducted for the US Department of Energy, for example, indicates that nearly 75% of cost overruns in the construction and operation of plants for new products and processes can be blamed on inadequate technical information.

Measurement and planning. Effective knowledge building is only the first step in improving returns from technical investments. The second step is to use this knowledge to plan better future investments. Armed with an understanding of the appropriate technical performance parameters, the limits alternative technical approaches place on these parameters, and an estimate of future R&D productivity based on analyses of past S-curves, senior management will be in a position to conduct a reasoned dialogue about the broad alternatives facing the company. In the course of this dialogue, existing assumptions grounded in conventional economic performance measures and incremental thinking are bound to be severely tested.

The ability to measure S-curve and R&D productivity can be integrated into the technical planning process to permit new assumptions to be tested. Then management can use these new technical information systems to determine which technology to pursue, when to pursue it, and at what levels of investment — and measure the results of these strategic decisions. Managers can determine whether a given effort has actually yielded the anticipated degree of performance improvement — and if not, why not. The conclusions, fed back into the technological planning and development process, can further refine its effectiveness. Such measures can rejuvenate a company.

Tuning in to Change

Radical technological change cuts away the company's base of technical and perhaps strategic intuition. Leading through the resulting maze of shifting organizational priorities requires new management priorities as well.

In most US corporations today, the CEO is the final arbiter of technological choice. It is he who finally decides to reallocate resources from old to new technologies. It is he who controls the pace of S-curve transitions, determining the rate of R&D funds transfer, the rate at which capital spending is shifted to new technologies, the redirection of marketing efforts — even the reallocation of managers.

The chief executive, in fact, *is* the corporate manager of technology. Unfortunately, the job is difficult. Confronted by an R&D program composed of dozens or hundreds of individual projects, small and large, the CEO is likely to be baffled by the task of assessing the relative value of each and relating it to the company's objectives, particularly in areas of rapid technological change. Yet if he cannot assure himself that R&D will be effectively focused on the technical alternatives with the greatest potential, he may be compromising the company's future.

The executive best qualified to aid the CEO is obviously the vice president in charge of R&D. But in too many US corporations this executive busies himself with more functional tasks — within boundaries implicitly set by the chief executive — than with basic issues of technological choice. In a recent Conference Board survey,[4] only one CEO in four named the R&D VP as a member of his inner circle. Something will need to change here. Until the R&D vice president earns the CEO's full confidence, strategic changes in technology will be painful, and future competitiveness in doubt.

Had such an executive been at Sylvania in the mid-1950s, he might have recruited more solid-state engineers. Were he in charge of R&D at a major chemical company today, he might be busy hiring biochemists, setting them up in an independent facility, and holding down investments in incremental improvement of conventional product or process technologies.

The R&D VP will need to become well tuned to overall competitive strategy and corporate options, and he may need to become more knowledgeable about corporate finance. He should establish a better working relationship with the top strategic planner and with the company's financial officers so that he can better empathize with their problems. In short, he will need to think like a CEO.

The Need to Anticipate

Since the shift to a new technology may take a decade or more to complete, most companies need to do a better job of anticipating technological development relatively far in advance. In short, they need a distant early warning capability.

In the mid-1930s, for example, Mervin Kelly, then research director of Bell Laboratories, projected telephone switching needs ahead to the early 1960s. He found that, with the current mechanical relay technology, an impossibly huge number of switches would be needed to support the future telephone network. This meant that a new technology would be needed. Kelly hypothesized that it might emerge from the new science of quantum mechanics. Accordingly, after World War II, he launched an R&D project to develop a quantum-mechanical amplifier. Bell Laboratories developed the first transistors in 1947; by 1955, transistors were an item of commerce. The whole process had taken 20 years (with 10 years out for the war).[5]

Development activities must be planned, funded, started, supported, and often completed before existing measurement systems can accurately predict their ultimate economic benefits for the company. But the rewards of anticipating future requirements are exceeded only by the costs of ignoring them.

One effective way a company can broaden its horizons is to push hard for the identification of technological alternatives. In the computer industry, for example, evidence is beginning to accumulate that solid-state components—designed and produced as they have been for the past 10 years—may be approaching the upper end of the S-curve. As the cost of creating ever more complex devices in the conventional way rises dramatically with each increment in performance, it is less and less economically feasible to persist with development at continually accelerating rates. Moreover, as the capacity of computer memories grows and the cost per bit of storage becomes infinitesimal, computer memories are becoming a commodity, and the market leverage of building bigger computers diminishes. This combination of increased expenditure needs and decreased leverage could create a scissors effect, constricting or even cutting off development. Already, in fact, the S-curve

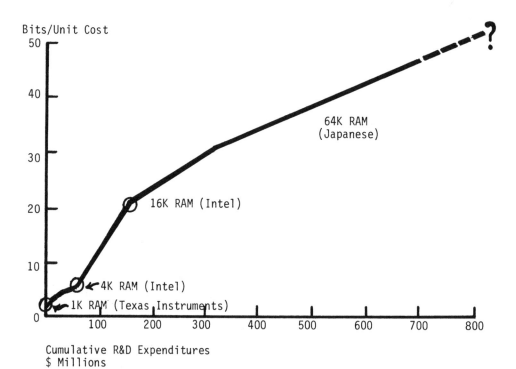

FIGURE 5. Topping Out in Electronic Hardware
Source: McKinsey analysis.

for random access memory chips (DRAMs) is exhibiting the classic phenomenon of diminishing returns (Figure 5), and many companies have already dropped out of the game.

As a result, it seems that the leverage in computer development is shifting from hardware to software, where no such diminishing returns are in sight. Monumental changes will accompany the transition. Manufacturing, always important in the computer hardware industry, may lose its place in the sun. Software manufacturers may already be beginning to embrace a strategy of creating only a few copies of each new design for distribution through telecommunications networks to the customers' own computers. With such an arrangement, the manufacturing process would take place, in a sense, on the customers' premises. The marketing manager would become a total business manager, controlling not only the sales of the product, but its manufacture and distribution as well.

Who would be most likely to survive such fundamental changes — the large hardware manufacturers, like IBM, Siemens, and Fujitsu, where manufacturing is an entrenched and powerful corporate function, or the smaller companies that now dominate the software industry? It may be hard to imagine anyone challenging IBM's preeminent position in the computer industry. But it was just as hard to imagine in 1955 that a little company called Texas Instruments would be a dominant force in electronics 10 years later. In the history of technological change, however, such revolutions are not rare. Companies that anticipate them, by continually investigating new alternatives and responding boldly to new challenges, are handsomely rewarded.

Notes

1. Robert W. Keyes, "Physical Limits in Semiconductor Electronics," *Science*, March 18, 1977, pp. 1230–1235.
2. McKinsey analysis based on industry interviews.
3. Merrow, E.W. *et al.*, "Understanding Cost Growth and Performance: Shortfalls in Pioneer Process Plants," RAND Corporation Report R-2569 (1981).
4. "Who Is Top Management?," The Conference Board, Report no. 821 (1982).
5. Based on conversations with Bell Laboratories executives. For more on the development of the transistor, see Jeremy Bernstein, *Three Degrees Above Zero* (New York: Charles Scribner's Sons, 1984), especially p. 119.

The Emergence of Technology Strategy
A New Dimension of Strategic Management
John Friar and Mel Horwitch

ABSTRACT. *This article deals with the rise and character of modern technology strategy. The current elevation of technology to a strategic variable is discussed, and the key forces behind this trend are identified. The current blending of two previously distinctive private-sector modes of innovation — small high-technology firm entrepreneurialism and large corporate industrial R&D — is highlighted. A conceptual framework, consisting of decisions and trade-offs along the three dimensions of competitive strategy, domain and structure, is given. Empirical support, based on both industry-level and firm-level data and analysis, is presented. It is argued that, over the past few years, the approaches used by corporations for developing and acquiring technology have become more numerous and varied with the relative significance increasing for internal decentralized entrepreneurial units and external approaches. A stabilization or consolidation of technology strategy approaches, however, may take place in the near future. Still, the emergence of modern technology strategy has permanently changed the landscape of the strategic management field.*

The real acceptance of technology's strategic importance is a relatively recent phenomenon. In the past, viewing technology as an essential part of corporate strategy was largely absent in strategic management thinking and practice.[1] The emergence of *technology strategy* today, however, is a significant, enduring and novel aspect of modern strategic management.

This article discusses the background, dimensions and implications of this elevation of technology to a strategic variable. A historical and conceptual overview is provided. Then the significant directions of technology strategy patterns are docu-

John Friar is finishing his Ph.D. dissertation on the relationship between technological advance and competitive advantage in the medical diagnostic equipment industry. He is a member of the Management of Technology and Strategy group at the Sloan School of Management, MIT. Mr. Friar received an MBA from the Harvard Business School, and has worked as director of marketing and planning for a division of North American Philips Corporation. His previous experience also includes engineering work on the Space Shuttle as an employee of Draper Laboratories.

Mel Horwitch is a member of the corporate planning, policy and strategy group at the Alfred P. Sloan School of Management, MIT. He has worked in both government and private industry, and has written extensively on strategic management, technology, energy affairs, and large-scale programs and projects. His most recent book is Clipped Wings: The American SST Conflict. *He is completing a book on modern strategic management.*

mented and analyzed at two levels: industry and firm. First, the relevant changing patterns in four very different kinds of technology-intensive industries are examined: personal computers, diagnostic ultrasound equipment, manufacturing technology, and biotechnology. Second, the technology strategy patterns in a number of large technology-intensive firms are analyzed. Finally, the implications of the ideas and findings in this article and an assessment of future directions for technology strategy are discussed.

Before discussing specifically the characteristics of modern technology strategy, the activity itself requires some further elaboration and explanation. Technology strategy can meaningfully be distinguished from other overlapping technology-related aspects of business behavior. Technological innovation traditionally has been portrayed largely as a subject separate from other management practices, including strategy. Technology has been studied in considerable depth as part of R&D management and the process of technological innovation; it has been reviewed as a determinant of organization structure; and it has been seen as being a critical factor in influencing the evolution of the international product life cycle.[2] Modern technological innovation, furthermore, is now recognized as a complex activity. One important aspect of our growing understanding is the realization that technological innovation is a process, made up of diverse parts, varied participants, complicated patterns of evolution and information feedback loops, and potentially lengthy time durations. Great emphasis is now placed on the roles of "market pull" and "user needs." Important research continues to highlight the key role of people, as champions, entrepreneurs, or technology-familiar managers, in effectively promoting and accelerating innovation.[3] Moreover, while such activities as R&D management, new product development, process improvement, or even overall technological innovation obviously form part of technology strategy, they do not usually encompass such key aspects of corporate strategy as top management involvement, high-level planning, and strategic resource allocation.

Both technology and strategy, moreover, are ambiguous concepts. "Technology" can be viewed as the ability to create a reproduceable way for generating improved products, processes and services. This capacity is both a formal and informal activity. Its result can be radical or incremental in nature. "Strategy" is probably an even more ambiguous term than technology. Definitions of strategy abound. As seen in Figure 1, however, there is general agreement that strategy involves the interplay and trade-offs of three sets of dimensions: present and future, internal and external considerations, and explicit (*e.g.*, formal) and implicit (*e.g.*, informal) managerial practices.

For much of the postwar period in the United States, technology and corporate strategy were distinctly separate fields and areas of activity. The key ingredients for technological vitality in industry appeared to be the vigorous functioning of different kinds of technological innovation and the active interplay of two distinctly separate forms of private-sector technological innovative activity — small-company and large-scale-corporation innovation.[4]

Corporate strategy as described above was usually not part of a small firm's management repertoire. Instead, strategy — if it related to technology anywhere — belonged to the realm of the large-scale corporation and, hence, its R&D activities. But even in this case, technology was not usually considered in truly strategic terms.

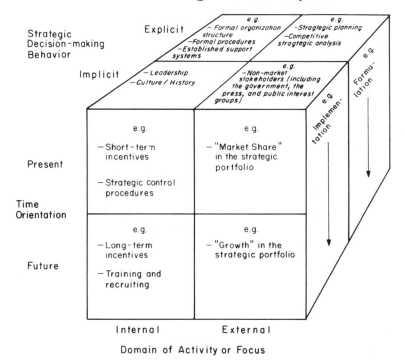

FIGURE 1. The dimensions of corporate strategy.

Technology strategy has a top-level and total-form perspective. It is, in essence, that set of activities by which management chooses its technological activity, allocates the resources for its technological undertakings, and structures the overall context for the development and maintenance of the technological resources that support the long-term strategic direction of a firm. Technology strategy has intimate ties with the other functional strategies of a corporation, including marketing, manufacturing, finance, and human resources. Moreover, it has a profound impact on the business strategies of a firm, such as in creating synergies between businesses, in extending or transforming the life cycles of various products, or in creating opportunities for forward and backward vertical integration.

Five Historical Forces

The recognition of technology as a top-level and strategic concern for a corporation was due to the convergence of at least five historical forces that, by the 1980s, had pushed technology to the fore.

The first element was a growing reaction to the seeming dominance of strategic planning that occurred during the preceding decade of the 1970s. This earlier period was a kind of "Golden Age" of strategic planning that was supported by strategic planning staffs within firms and a network of information and analysis industries and institutions that included strategic consulting firms, business schools, and strategic-level, computer-based models. To a greater or lesser degree, much of the center of gravity in strategic management shifted from an earlier tradition in strategic management that had emphasized such imprecise and informal general management factors as leadership, interpersonal skills, experience, and vision to the seemingly more rigorous, objective and formal standards associated with strategic planning. Intense international competition increased, however, with foreign competitors succeeding apparently without the help of strategic planning staffs or consultants. Moreover, previous assumptions associated with strategic planning, such as the universal benefits of large market share, were questioned. Consequently, strategic planning came under attack. It was increasingly seen as possibly a costly piece of overhead. As corporations began to reconsider the process of creating real wealth or value, they turned toward technology as a key vehicle for accomplishing this goal.[5]

A second source of the intensifying interest in technology as a strategic weapon was the obvious success of small high-technology firms in a host of emerging technology-intensive industries, such as instruments, semiconductors, computers and software. Here was another model for creating new wealth, neither dependent upon strategic planning staffs and consultants nor upon huge industrial R&D facilities and units. Instead, the key ingredients for success appeared to be risk-taking, technological champions and entrepreneurs, intense commitment, informal and fluid organization structures, and fast response to changing market conditions. Some large corporations, like Hewlett-Packard and 3M, successfully incorporated many of these attributes into their own management systems and cultures. By the 1980s, other large firms were attempting—not necessarily successfully—the same thing at the expense of strategic planning and industrial R&D.[6] Again, this attention to new ways of organizing for innovation tended to raise the level and priority of technological decisions and deliberations in the corporation, often to the strategic level.

A third source that tended to promote technology as a strategic variable was the obviously high priority given to technology by the foreign competitors of US firms, particularly the Japanese. The growing importance of developing new technology in the corporate strategy of Japanese firms was increasingly recognized in the US. MITI openly admitted that its future lay in higher value-added industries and technological innovation.[7] As one Japanese scholar observed, by the late 1970s, with the successful completion of MITI's dramatic and significant VSLI Project in semiconductors, Japan moved from imitation to innovation.[8] Eventually, by the early 1980s, the sheer impact of the acknowledged Japanese successes in such technology-intensive global industries as robotics, semiconductors, computers, telecommunications and ceramics would alone raise the role of technology in US firms to a high level of significance.[9]

A fourth element that increased the visibility of technology was the concurrent rise in status and importance of manufacturing as a strategic weapon. During the 1960–1980 period, the competitive role of manufacturing had diminished in the US. Two main trends were responsible for this decline in the strategic use of manufacturing by American management. First, the manufacturing function increasingly became a subsidiary activity in the corporation. It grew more and more technical, and was often equated with the more discipline-based concerns of operations research. Moreover, the main purpose of manufacturing — or operations management, as this field was increasingly termed — was, more often than not, to fine-tune the task of mass production. The strategic role of manufacturing until the decade of the 1980s was largely ignored.

But, again triggered especially by effective foreign competition, the key strategic significance of such manufacturing considerations as flexibility, quality, rapid change-overs, and process trade-offs was increasingly recognized. Moreover, the concurrent incorporation of new electronic and information technologies into manufacturing (which resulted in new capabilities for manufacturing operations, and altered the meaning of traditional experience-curve and operations management concepts) also accelerated the rediscovery of manufacturing as a strategic weapon. By the early 1980s, the lonely cries of a decade earlier for a broader and more elevated view of manufacturing were finally echoed with increasing frequency, intensity and support.

Significantly, those calling for an enhanced place for manufacturing issued similar pleas for technology. In fact, it is somewhat surprising and ironical that the calls for giving technology a strategic role initially emanated more from the strategic wing of the manufacturing area than from the management of technology field itself.[10]

The final element that gave impetus to the rise of technology as a strategic variable was the force of ongoing research and thinking in the fields of strategic management and the management of technology. In the former area, in spite of the apparent victory of the formal and technocratic methodology represented by strategic planning, the older general management tradition had by no means vanished. By the end of the 1970s, as the vulnerability of strategic planning became increasingly apparent, the value of the lessons from the older general management approach was once again acknowledged, and new research rediscovered this perspective. Works emphasizing leadership, implementation, corporate culture, and a return to fundamentals were once more widely embraced.[11] Practically all such strategic thinking stressed the importance of innovation. Simultaneously, within the management of technology field, a base of knowledge and concepts was developed. Technology was increasingly seen as important and often critical to the whole firm. A dissatisfaction with the traditional fragmentation and the narrow specialties of this field took place. There were calls for a broad firm-level synthesis of the management of technology area, which tended to become strategic in perspective.[12]

By the early 1980s, the full impact of these five historical forces — the negative reaction to strategic planning, the success of the small high-technology firm, the increasingly strategic importance allocated to technology by foreign competition (particularly the Japanese), the related rise in status of manufacturing as a strategic weapon, and the supportive relevant thinking and research in the fields of strategic management and the management of technology — was visible, widespread, and powerful. Technology strategy has become an important management activity in the corporation.

Major Characteristics

What are the major characteristics of this phenomenon, termed technology strategy, that emerged in the early 1980s? In order to discuss this issue, both a historical and a conceptual view are required.

A historical perspective is important for recognizing just how fundamental the current transformation, represented by the rise of technology strategy, is. In fact, there has been a strategic blending of two earlier paradigms for private-sector technological innovation: small high-technology firm entrepreneurship and large-scale corporate innovation. Through approximately the 1970s (as seen in Figure 2), private-sector US technological innovation could logically be viewed as comprising two paradigms or ideal types: 1) Mode I—small high-technology firm entrepreneurship; and 2) Mode II—large-scale corporation R&D.[13] Mode I might well be designated the "Silicon Valley Model" of innovation. It represented a fundamentally new and

Key Mode Attributes	Inputs				Internal Processes			Output
Important Modes of Tech. Innovation	Technology/ Skills Available	Environment	Market	Goal Setting	Communication System	Organization Structure		Innovation: Product Line or Process or Systems
MODE I*	-emphasis on exploiting existing & known technologies -technological capabilities restricted to few areas -key technological skills reside in top management	-contained & definable	-markets for the product are few & definable	-goals are set by top man -goal-setting is informal with few actors involved -options open to the firm are few	-informal -few people -dissemination of information does not demand complex system due to few recipients	-organization -structure emphasizes few sub-units & informality -top management gets involved in all activities in the organization		-typically a product or a product-line scope tends to be limited by the technological capabilities of the top management
MODE II**	-complex in defined product or process areas -skills consist of technological as well as non-technological, line marketing, in these areas. Mode II is concerned with existing & non-existing technologies which they help to develop	-multiple & complex but still definable	-markets for innovations are multi-user markets & complex	-innovation goals are partially set by formal systems -firm has several technological options to choose from -top management may or may not be directly involved in identifying or pursuing technological options	-complex due to several organizational levels, formal & informal communication is possible but difficult to achieve	-organization tends to be complex, divided into product groups, divisions, etc. -often different sub-units have conflicting attitude & priorities -corporate boundaries are definable		-large number and/or complex products & processes

Source: Mel Horwitch, "The Blending of Two Paradigms for Private-Sector Technology Strategy" in Jerry Dermer, ed., Competitiveness Through Technology: What Business Needs from Government (Lexington, MA: Lexington Books, Inc., forthcoming).

*Technological innovation process in small, entrepreneurial, high-technology firms.
**Technological innovation in large, multi-product, multi-market and/or multi-divisional corporations.

FIGURE 2. A comparison of the characteristics of the two modes of private-sector technological innovation.

dramatic phenomenon in American business history, where highly trained and well-educated technological entrepreneurs, during the period from the 1950s through the 1970s, created small high-technology firms in regions known for high-quality universities, such as Silicon Valley in California, Route 128 in the Boston area, the Research Triangle in North Carolina, and Route 1 near Princeton, New Jersey.[14]

The salient features of Mode I included: a strong commitment generally to a single, narrow or focused technology area; a comparatively small, informal and changing organizational structure; a technological champion as head of the firm or part of the top-management team; and an overall climate and style of entrepreneurship and risk-taking. The key frequent weaknesses of Mode I organizations were also apparent: an absence of basic business skills, the huge and sometimes negative role that the personality traits of the founder could play, a lack of various kinds of resources, and the dependence usually on a single technology or product-market area.

Co-existing with Mode I firms and even pre-dating them were Mode II corporations and the traditional technological innovation process within them. Technological innovation in the Mode II multi-division, multi-product and multi-market context often presented a generally different set of behavior patterns and challenges than those found in a typical Mode I environment. The major managerial problems for Mode II technological innovation through the 1970s, as seen in Figure 3, usually included making strategic choices or trade-offs along at least three sets of dimensions: types of technological innovation, the specific technologies to develop, and the timing or positioning of technology introduction into the marketplace (in Figure 3, Freeman's classification terminology for this last dimension is employed — offensive, defensive, imitative, dependent, traditional and opportunist — but other classification schemes may be equally appropriate).[15]

Even after strategic decisions are more or less established, the Mode II corporation still had to deal with a number of complex internal strategic activities, including technological resource allocation, monitoring and evaluation of technological undertakings, the design of an appropriate structure, the location of the innovating activity, internal technology transfer, and the relationship between the early R&D work, the developmental work, and the operating divisions. The linkages between technological innovation activity and ongoing and pervasive formal procedures represented a particularly important difference between Mode II and Mode I environments. Similarly, the significant and often novel opportunities for technological synergies were also a major aspect of Mode II technological innovation.

A glaring weakness that was often attributed to traditional Mode II conditions was the absence of crucial entrepreneurial and risk-taking behavior patterns that were associated with Mode I. Cultivating and maintaining such behavior in the large corporation has become a major challenge for modern technology strategy. Although this earlier postwar paradigm of private-sector technological innovation involved the separate functioning, co-existence and interplay of two distinctive modes of technological innovation, effective and vigorous Mode I-like behavior was increasingly viewed as important for most successful innovations, even in a Mode II context.

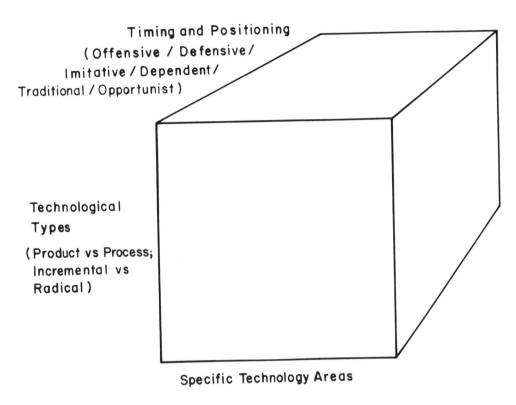

FIGURE 3. Mode II concepts for technological strategic choices through the 1970s.

Source: Mel Horwitch, "The Blending of Two Paradigms for Private-Sector Technology Strategy" in Jerry Dermer, ed., Competitiveness Through Technology: What Business Needs from Government (Lexington, MA: Lexington Books, Inc., forthcoming).

Fading Boundaries

By the early 1980s, as technology became increasingly strategic, the boundary between the two major forms of private-sector technological innovative activity—small-firm and large-corporation innovation—began to fade. This blending of these previously distinctive modes is a salient feature of modern technology strategy.[16] Small technology-intensive firms are becoming increasingly "professional" in managerial practices. They are savvy about the capital markets, and can negotiate effectively with large firms. Meanwhile, large corporations are increasingly attempting to install within their organizations and cultures Mode I structures and behavior. The previous separation no longer holds. Out of this fundamental blending, modern technology strategy has emerged. Now a complex array of trade-offs, relationships and linkages has to be managed. In order to better understand this new situation, a conceptual framework is helpful, and is presented in Figure 4.

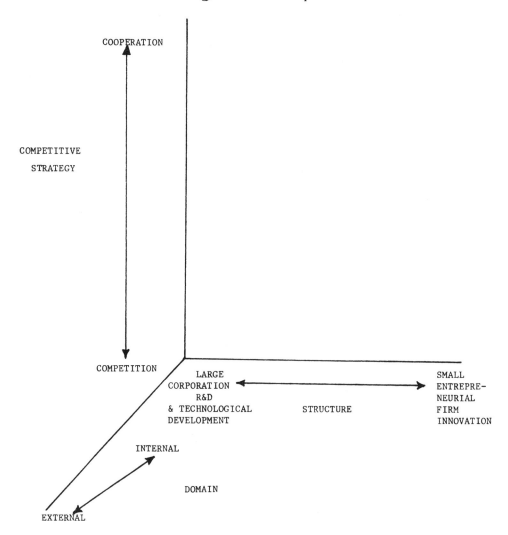

FIGURE 4. Elements of modern technology strategy.

Large modern technology-intensive corporations are making technology strategy decisions along three dimensions: competition vs. cooperation (competitive strategy); internal vs. external development (domain); and traditional R&D organizations, *e.g.*, the industrial R&D facility, vs. decentralized entrepreneurial units (structure).

Achieving the appropriate set of multiple trade-offs along these dimensions is one of the major tasks in technology strategy today, but it does not necessarily lead to making simple choices.

To take but one example related especially to the dimension of structure, recent research, based on the multi-business-unit PIMS database, has uncovered many distinctive kinds of technology-intensive businesses.[17] Seven were identified. Four are in the industrial products area (Established Suppliers, Fast Movers, High-Tech Job Shops, and Stalled Giants), and three are in the consumer products area (Established Diversifiers, Dominant Specialists, and Laggers). Moreover, focusing on the intra-organizational linkages of vertical integration, shared facilities, or shared marketing, a complex group of success patterns was found. Success was found to depend upon the type of technology-intensive business, the criteria for success (in this case, market share or ROI), and structure. Clearly, designing a sound structure for effective technology strategy involves more, for example, than merely possessing or trading off mainstream industrial R&D and decentralized venture units.

The Emergence of Modern Technology Strategy: An Industry-Level Perspective

In order to document more fully the extent and dimensions of modern technology strategy, two types of information will be presented. First, a brief review of representative technology-intensive industries will be given. Second, an analysis of the technology strategies of representative large US technology-intensive corporations will be made.

Personal Computers

The personal computer industry, one of the clearest examples of an entrepreneurially launched technology-intensive industry, illustrates on a macro level the current transition of technology strategy. In the latter half of the 1970s, the true spark for this industry came from an entrepreneurial small-firm environment that was made up of hobbyists, publicists and promoters, technological champions, and entrepreneurs.[18] As seen in Table 1, all three of the major initial start-up firms in the personal computer industry, MITS, IMSAI and Processor Technology, failed in the marketplace, and did not create sustainable businesses. Although they were very

TABLE 1. Market share (by dollar sales) of the US personal computer industry

Company	1976	1978	1980	1982
MITS	25%			
IMSAI	17%			
Processor Technology	8%			
Radio Shack		50%	21%	10%
Commodore International		12%	20%	12%
Apple		10%	27%	26%
IBM				17%
NEC			5%	11%
Hewlett-Packard			9%	7%
Other	50%	28%	18%	17%
Total	100%	100%	100%	100%
Total Units	15,000	200,000	500,000	1,500,000

Sources: Gary N. Farner, *A Competitive Analysis of the Personal Computer Industry*, MIT, Alfred P. Sloan School of Management, unpublished Master's Thesis, May 20, 1982, p. 18. Deborah F. Schreiber, *The Strategic Evolution of the Personal Computer Industry*, MIT, Alfred P. Sloan School of Management, unpublished Master's Thesis, May, 1983, p. 7.

different kinds of firms, these early personal computer firms in different ways often lacked certain essential business skills. Their fates also frequently hinged on some counter-productive personality traits of the founding entrepreneurs.

But there was an important "second wave" in the early personal computer industry, beginning with the appearance in 1977–1978 of one totally new firm, Apple, and two large, established firms that entered from other industries, Radio Shack-Tandy and Commodore International. All three firms entered the personal computer industry at about the same time. For different reasons, all three were successful.

Apple reflected the best of small-firm behavior: an innovative and adaptable technology and product design, skilled technological champions at the top, a strong entrepreneurial drive, and a remarkably effective, informal and spirited organization. Radio Shack-Tandy had a good product design, excellent service and support, and a superb marketing and distribution system. Commodore International had good marketing and low-cost production through vertical integration.

During this "second wave," small and large computer firms remained more or less distinct. But there was a vital interplay between them as people flowed from one firm to another, and with this flow, the transfer of technology and relevant managerial knowledge and technique took place. There was co-existence, but separateness.

But the traditional small firm/large firm dichotomy appears to have broken down in personal computers. As indicated in Table 1, a dramatic development in the industry occurred with the entrance of IBM. The firm quickly captured a huge market share, particularly in the business market. In June 1984, a sample survey of 37 *Fortune* 500 companies found that 95% had as primary personal computer hardware IBM, PC, PC/XT, or PC-compatible machines.[19]

Much of IBM's market success in personal computers lies in the novel way IBM structured itself to enter the personal computer industry. The firm went outside its mainstream R&D processes to establish an Independent Business Unit (IBU) to develop personal computers. The IBU worked separately from the rest of IBM, and created, for IBM, a non-traditional product and product strategy. The IBM PC uses off-the-shelf components and an outside operating system, MS-DOS. Also, its operating system architecture is open, so that third parties can develop software. Moreover, instead of solely selling through its own sales force, IBM also sells PCs through retail outlets.[20]

On another front, in August 1983, IBM boosted its equity position in Intel, its key PC microprocessor supplier, to about 13.7%. Rather than just making a good financial investment, IBM appeared to be taking strategic action to protect its and America's technological base by strengthening a key US innovator.[21] IBM had both created a small-firm-like organization within its overall large-corporation structure, and had established a number of novel external linkages.

More generally, as indicated in Figure 5, the personal computer industry has witnessed an increasing number of key strategic linkages that spans types of technological innovation, countries, and organizations. AT&T has bought 25% of Olivetti, and Olivetti quickly designed and produced an IBM-compatible machine for AT&T to sell, beginning in July 1984. AT&T also has contracted with Convergent Technologies, a small firm in the Silicon Valley, to develop and produce a Unix-based PC.[22] Meanwhile, the Japanese ceramics firm, Kyocera, has built highly successful lap computers for Radio Shack-Tandy, NEC and Olivetti.[23]

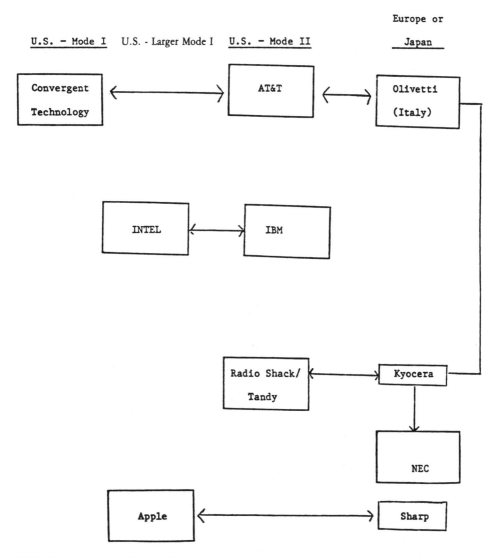

FIGURE 5. A selected list of linkages in the personal computer industry, 1983–1984.

Sources: Various Issues of InfoWorld in 1983 and 1984.

Finally, Apple now has Sharp making its flat LCD display for its trim IIc computer. Apple also markets Canon's new laser printer in the United States, while Canon markets Apple's MacIntosh computer in Japan. Both firms are working on software for the MacIntosh for the Japanese market.[24]

Diagnostic Ultrasound Equipment

The medical electronic equipment industry can be divided into five broad segments: diagnostic, monitoring, therapeutic, prosthetic, and surgical support.[25] The medical electronic equipment market in the US was estimated at $3.7 billion in 1983 with the diagnostic segment, which comprises about 350 US firms, accounting for 45% of that total. Worldwide sales of the entire industry are estimated to be twice that of US sales, so the worldwide market was about $7.4 billion in 1983. The worldwide market is estimated to be growing at 15–20% annually, although some of the subsegments are growing at twice that rate.

In many ways, this industry is the prototypical high-technology industry. Because the markets are large and growing rapidly, many firms have entered the industry. Entry barriers are low. Manufacturing consists of component assembly, with components typically comprising 85% of the cost of the equipment. So manufacturing value-added is very low. Distribution and service can be provided by manufacturers' representatives until a firm reaches a scale to perform direct sales. Capital has been available from venture capitalists, although high levels are not needed, because the research costs are often bootlegged from large firms, universities, and government research groups. Many new firms are divisions of companies not originally in the medical electronic equipment industry. They have used expertise from other fields to enter these markets.

The product value-added that a company can provide is in its proprietary assemblage of common components. This ability, however, is readily duplicated and hard to defend.

No single company markets products in all major categories of equipment, although some companies emphasize breadth of product line. No company, moreover, dominates any single product line, because no company has been able to transfer product-line dominance across countries.

The industry, then, appears to be highly fragmented with the number of firms still growing. The industry is not one that is likely to go through the well-known cycle of birth, growth, maturation and decay. Continued product technology advancements, both major and incremental, are expected. A dramatic shake-out of the industry, then, is highly unlikely.

But the strategic significance of inter-firm linkages in this seemingly hyper-fluid industry is high. Let us take, for example, a segment of this industry, diagnostic ultrasound. About 80 companies now compete in diagnostic ultrasound. The top five companies held less than 50% of the market in 1980. More new companies are expected to enter, and the drive to constantly improve the technology is likely to continue.

Still, perhaps because of this constant churning, strategic linkages are crucial, as seen in Figure 6. Advances in the state of the art are considered to have come mostly from small, start-up companies, but even these companies have acquired technology from external sources. ATL started with technology it licensed from the University of Washington; Hoffrell, from the University of Pittsburgh; Unirad, from Battelle; and Diasonics, from Searle and Hitachi. Small companies, moreover, have acquired other companies for their technologies, such as Diasonics' acquisition of Varian and Fischer's acquisition of EMI Ultrasound.

Large companies have also used diverse avenues to enter and to develop various ultrasound technology segments. An example is General Electric. GE entered the ultrasound market by first hiring people away from Litton, and then selling a product originally developed by Litton and modified by Xonics. The rest of GE's prod-

GEC, Ltd.

Acquired Picker
Acquired Cambridge Instruments
Licensee of SRI and Hitachi.

General Electric

Bought technology from Electra-Physics (Litton) and
    hired Litton people.
B-scan product modified by Xonics
Linear array developed by Yokogawa
Phased array developed by Analogic Corporation
Mechanical sector developed by Second Foundation

Johnson & Johnson

Acquired Technicare (Ohio Nuclear, Unirad, Scientific
    Advances, Battelle)
Acquired Irex (Joint venture with Hoffrell)

Philips

Acquired Rohe Ultrasound (sold Kretz equipment)
Licensee of Matsushita
Supplied by Hoffrell

Siemens

Sold Diasonics equipment in Europe
Acquired Searle's line
Licensee of Matsushita

SmithKline

Started as joint venture with General Precision
    Corporation
Acquired rights to mechanical sector from Indianapolis
    Center for Advanced Research
Licensee of Mediscan (licensed Xerox)
Formed SKI and sold 80% to Xonics

Squibb

Acquired ATL (Licensee of Univ. of Washington and SRI)
Acquired ADR (Start-up from Unirad)

Diasonics

Start-up from Searle
Acquired Varian
Licensee of Hitachi
Joint development with Hitachi

Toshiba

Supplied to Litton
Hired Litton people

Hoffrell

Licensee of University of Pittsburgh
Licensor to Philips and Cambridge Instruments (Picker)
Joint venture with Irex (Johnson & Johnson)

Fischer

Acquired EMI

Unirad

Acquired by Ohio Nuclear and Technicare (Johnson & Johnson)

Xonics

Owns 80% of SKI (SmithKline)
Developed product for GE

Litton

Spawned G.E. and provided B-scan
Spawned Toshiba; original licensee of Toshiba

Searle

Spawned Diasonics
Acquired by Siemens

FIGURE 6. Technology linkages in the US diagnostic ultrasound industry, 1977–1982.

uct line was developed by Analogic Corporation, Yokogowa, and Second Foundation. GE has competed in ultrasound, then, by using outside technology to enter the product markets and by using internal development to create some further advances.

Other large corporations have used acquisitions to enter: Squibb acquired ATL and ADR; Philips acquired Rohe; Johnson & Johnson acquired Technicare. Along with GE, several firms are licensees of Japanese technology: Philips, Diasonics, Picker and Siemens. Joint ventures for the development of technology have also been evident; two examples are SmithKline with General Precision Corporation and Diasonics with Hitachi. Finally, large firms have taken equity positions in smaller firms, *e.g.*, SmithKline's 20% control of SKI, to maintain linkages with firms performing ultrasound technology development.

The diagnostic ultrasound industry, therefore, is characterized by a rich and varied technology-strategy environment. In 1985, about 80 companies competed in this segment. Many small start-up firms were vying for market share against large corporations. But both the small firms and the large corporations are using a broad range of techniques to develop and to acquire technology, including strategic linkages. Even in an apparently fluid technology-intensive setting, a blending of previously distinctive modes is taking place.

The Manufacturing Technology Industry

The same pattern of an evolving set of complex technology strategies is now manifested in the manufacturing technology industry, an industry with little of the postwar small-firm entrepreneurial experience that was part of the personal computer or diagnostic ultrasound equipment industries.

The US machine tool industry played an important and venerable role in US technological development and business history. During the latter half of the 19th century, the machine tool industry served as the vital link for developing and transferring technology to American industry as a whole.[26] But by the mid-20th century, the US machine tool sector was clearly in a mature phase, and had lost much of the technological vitality and importance as a salient industry that had characterized it in an earlier era.

In the postwar period until about 1980, this industry was not very glamorous or exciting from the point of view of technology strategy.[27] Defined as "power-driven machines, not hand held, that are used to cut, form or shape metal," the machine tool industry itself is a relatively small sector of the US economy, comprising about 0.12% of the GNP and 0.10% of the US employment in 1982. Most US machine tool firms have traditionally been small, closely held companies with narrow product lines. The industry is not highly concentrated with the four largest firms in 1977 accounting for 22% of industry shipments. Both sales and, to a lesser extent, employment are highly cyclical. Research and development expenses, capital investment outlays, and growth and productivity are all relatively low.

In 1982, in constant dollars, R&D expenses declined to about the same level that they were in 1975. The global market share of the US machine tool industry decreased from 25% in 1968 to 20% or less in the 1970s. In terms of both growth and productivity, the US machine tool industry during the 1973–1981 period fell way behind US manufacturing as a whole, and, in the case of productivity, behind durable goods manufacturing. During the postwar period, until perhaps very recently, the US machine tool industry generally exhibited a short-term outlook, concerned mostly with annual financial goals.

The US machine tool sector, therefore, seemed to resemble the prototypical "smokestack" or "sunset" industry. Under the impact of effective global competition and the apparent failure to exploit or keep up with various new technologies in manufacturing, such as new materials, software, CAD/CAM and automation, the US machine tool firms have become progressively less profitable, and have lost significant market share. Moreover, there was generally an absence of significant small-firm innovation activity with the possible exception of the robotics field.[28] Even in robotics, however, much of the technological leadership during the 1970s shifted to Japanese companies. In addition, the relatively large US firms also did not generally exhibit significant technological R&D activity or leadership. In machine tools during the 1970s, there was very little of the creative and vital interplay between distinctly small-firm and large-firm innovation that was manifested, for example, in the "second wave" of the early personal computer industry. Instead, the US machine tool industry stagnated, and various global competitors took quick advantage of this situation.

But such a gloomy picture of machine tools actually needs revision today. If the definition of machine tools is broadened to encompass manufacturing process technology as a whole, rather than just metal-bending or metal-cutting, then the industry is now clearly experiencing a major restructuring. The development of software, CAD/CAM, robots, systems and, ultimately, full-scale factory automation is dramatically changing what had seemed to be a stagnant, sunset industry into a technologically vigorous one that possesses some of the new patterns of technology strategy manifested in more stereotypical modern technology-intensive industries. As seen in Figure 7, the industry is becoming more complex in terms of proliferating "strategic groups,"[29] and is attracting a wide array of new entrants, ranging from new, small, high-technology firms to established large manufacturing firms like General Electric, Westinghouse and IBM.[30]

The current pattern of technology strategy in the manufacturing process technology industry, therefore, also exhibits an increasing blurring of the various distinctive types of technological innovation and a growing profusion of linkages between types of innovation and between firms.

These trends can be seen by focusing on one strategic group within the whole manufacturing process technology industry, robotics.[31] The overall American effort to develop robotics until about 1980 was fragmented, limited to a few players, and lacked the support of crucial stakeholders, such as large industrial concerns and the government. As seen in Figure 8, until very recently, practically all robotics activity in the US was concentrated in a few companies with two firms, Unimation and Cincinnati Milacron, together accounting for greater than 50% of the US market share through 1982. Like machine tools, robotics in the US was in the industrial R&D backwater, and, except for Cincinnati Milacron and a few small firms, was largely a low-priority R&D item until the 1980s. The involvement of large manu-

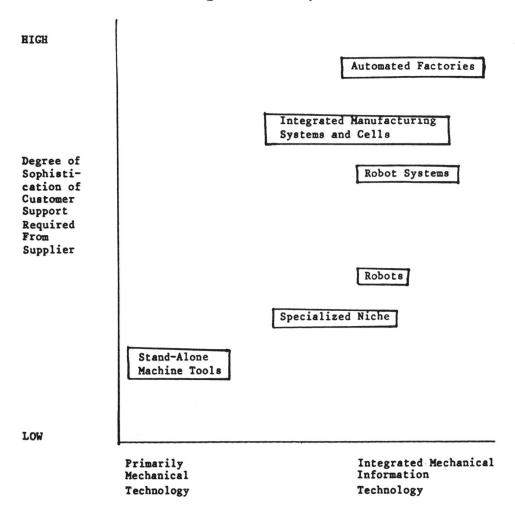

FIGURE 7. Strategic groups in the manufacturing technology industry.
Source: National Research Council, *The U.S. Machine Tool Industry and the Defense Industrial Base* (Washington, D.C.: National Academy Press, 1983).

facturing enterprises and corporations with strong capabilities in the key technologies and frequently with huge captive markets was practically non-existent until the 1980s.

By 1980, however, the situation was beginning to change. The growth rate of US robotics sales was accelerating, and — just as significant — important new entrants had appeared. The new entrants, as seen in Table 2, were not primarily new start-up ventures. Instead, they represented large established enterprises with strong manufacturing and technological skills.

Large and small firms are now fully represented. A technology-based industry

(Symbols in Parentheses Indicate Mode of Innovation)

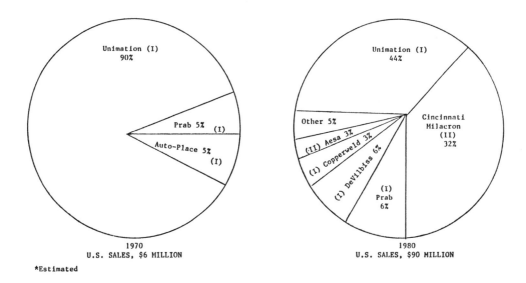

FIGURE 8. US robotics industry sales and market share.
Source: L. Conigliaro, *Robotics Newsletter*, Number 9, Bache Halsey Stuart Shield, Inc., 1982; and modified by authors.

is now on the verge of a probable take-off. Figure 9 shows that, at some point in the early 1980s, the rate of growth of the US robotics industry began to increase significantly.

In addition, as seen in Figure 10, suddenly a whole, rich array of linkages, many of which are international in character, is being established through licensing agreements, joint ventures, and mergers and acquisitions. A new complex set of technology-strategy patterns now exists in the US robotics industry, perhaps just in time.

The Biotechnology Industry

The biotechnology industry is still another type of technology-based industry.[32] It is young and global. Almost from the start, it has possessed a full set of complex strategic relationships. All forms of modern technology strategy are represented in this sector, as seen in Figure 11.

The major US small firms, such as Genentech, Biogen and Cetus, have equity and/or research linkages with several large corporations throughout the world. A number of major large corporations, such as Eli Lilly, Monsanto and—to a more limited degree—DuPont, in addition to sizeable internal R&D activity, are actively linked in diverse ways with other firms. In fact, these intertwining relationships are global in nature, as seen in Figure 12, which illustrates US-Japanese strategic connections.

TABLE 2. Market Share: U.S. based robot vendors (1980–1983)

	1980	1981	1982	1983
Unimation	44.4%	43.8%	32.1%	22.8%
Cincinnati Milacron	32.2%	32.2%	21.0%	16.2%
DeVilbiss	5.5%	4.2%	7.4%	6.7%
Asea Inc.	2.8%	5.8%	8.7%	7.2%
Prab Robots Inc.	6.1%	5.3%	4.2%	4.2%
Cybotech	—	—	1.4%	2.3%
Copperweld Robotics	3.3%	2.3%	2.3%	1.8%
Automatix	0.4%	1.9%	4.2%	7.6%
Advanced Robotics Corp.	1.9%	0.5%	3.5%	3.2%
Mordson	0.8%	1.6%	2.5%	2.5%
Thermwood	—	0.6%	1.6%	1.4%
Bendix	—	—	1.4%	2.3%
GCA Industrial Systems	—	—	1.0%	2.9%
IBM	—	—	0.7%	3.0%
GE	—	—	0.9%	1.1%
Westinghouse	—	—	0.4%	1.5%
U.S. Robots	—	—	0.6%	1.5%
Graco	—	—	0.6%	1.5%
Mobot	0.9%	0.4%	0.8%	0.8%
GM/Fanuc	—	—	1.5%	3.0%
American Robot	—	—	—	0.6%
Textron	—	—	—	0.3%
Nova Robotics	—	—	—	0.3%
Control Automation	—	—	0.1%	0.3%
Machine Intelligence	—	—	—	1.1%
Intelledex	—	—	—	0.6%
Other	1.7%	1.3%	1.5%	1.7%
	100.0%	100.0%	100.0%	100.0%

SOURCE: L. Conigliaro, *Robotics Newsletter*, Number 9, Bache Halsey Stuart Shield, Inc., 1982.

The Emergence of Modern Technology Strategy: A Firm-Level Perspective

The companies selected for our firm-level analysis of modern technology strategy were from those US-based *Fortune* 500 companies that had spent at least $80 million on R&D in 1982, as listed by *Business Week* (March 21, 1984). It was assumed that companies which had spent this much money on R&D had large R&D organizations extant with the capabilities to initiate a complex set of research projects. Furthermore, these firms would also be able to locate and acquire technical skills that were not presently in-house.

Given the apparently huge capability of such firms, the selection criteria for the companies to be studied was purposely biased toward firms that *a priori*, if possible, would want to keep as much of their technology development under direct control.

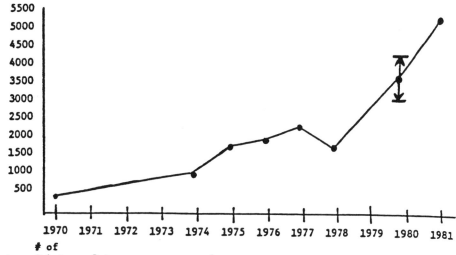

Point	# of Robots	Date	Source
A	200	1970 (April)	Engelberger, First National Symposium on Industrial Robots, 1970
B	1200	1974 (Dec.)	Frost and Sullivan, U.S. Industrial Robot Market, 1974
C	2000	1975 (Dec.)	Frost and Sullivan, The Industrial Robot Market in Europe, 1975
D	2000	1976 (Dec.)	Eikonix Technology Assessment, 1979
E	2400	1977 (Dec.)	Eikonix Technology Assessment, 1979
F	1600	1978 (Dec.)	American Machinist 12th Inventory, 1978
G	3000	1980 (Jan.)	Walt Weisel, Prab Conveyors
H	3500	1980 (June)	Business Week, Verfied by Cincinnati Milacron
I	3200	1980 (Dec.)	General Motors Technical Staff, (Bache, Shields estimate)
J	4000	1980 (Dec.)	Walt Weisel, Prab Conveyors
K	5500	1981 (Dec.)	Seiko Inc., Marketing Dept.

FIGURE 9. Estimates of US robot population, 1970–1981.

SOURCE: David Schatz, <u>The Strategic Evolution of the Robotics Industry</u> Unpublished Master's Thesis, Sloan School, MIT, May 1983.

LICENSING AGREEMENTS

Licensee	Licensor
Kawasaki Heavy Ind. (Japan)	Unimation
RN Eurobotics (Belgium)	Arab
Can-Eng. Mfg. (Canada)	"
Murata Machinery (Japan)	"
Binks (U.K.)	Thermwood
Cyclomatic Ind.	"
Didde Graphics Co.	"
DeVilbiss	Trallfa (Norway)
Nordson	Taskawa (Japan)
Admiral Equip. Co.	"
Bendix	
Automatix	Hitachi (Japan)
General Electric	"
Interred	"
Graco	Nolaug (Norway)
United Technologies	Nimak (W. Germany)
RCA	Dainichi Kiko (Japan)
I.B.M.	Sankyo Seiki (Japan)
General Electric	DEA (Italy)
" "	Volkswagen (W. Germany)
Westinghouse	Olivetti (Italy)
"	Hisubishi Electric (Japan)
"	Komatsu (Japan)
	Jobs Robots (Italy)
Lloyd Tool and Mfg.	

JOINT VENTURES

J.V.	Parents
Unimation	Condac, Pullman Corp.
GMF Robotics, Inc.	General Motors, Fanuc
Cybotech	Renault, Randsburg
	Industries
Int'l. Machine Intell.	Machine Intelligence,
Int'l. Machine Intell.	Yaskawa
Graco Robotics	Graco Inc., Edon Finishing

MERGERS AND ACQUISITIONS

Subsidiary	Parent
Unimation	Westinghouse
PAR Systems	GCA
U.S. Robots	Square D. Corp.
Copperweld Robotics	Copperweld Corp.
(formerly Auto-Place)	

FIGURE 10. Interfirm linkages in the US robotics industry, 1983.
Source: David Schatz, *The Strategic Evolution of the Robotics Industry*, Unpublished Master's Thesis, Sloan School, MIT, May 1983.

Important modes of Technological Innovation \ Home Countries of firms	United States	Japan	France	Other
Small Firm	Genentech, Cetus, Collaborative Res., Genex, Bethesda Res. Labs, Agrigenetics, Hybritech, Molecular Genetics, Calgene, Amgen, Collagen, Eugenics, Inten'l Plant Res. Inst., Genetics Institute	There are several small biotechnology firms in Japan, including Hayashibara Biochemical, Wakunaga Pharmaceutical		Biogen (Swiss & U.S.), Novo Industrie (Den.), Fortia (Sweden)
Large Corporation	Du Pont, Campbell Soup, Monsanto, Johnson & Johnson, Eli Lilly, Fluor, Corning Glass, Amoco, Socal, Chevron, Exxon, Nat. Distillers Corp., Upjohn, Pfizer, Searle, Merck, Mobil Oil, Allied, Koppers, Dennison, Bristol Myers, Dow Chemical, Phillips, Phillips Petrol., Occidental Petroleum (Zoecon), DeKalb, Agresearch, ARCO, GE, Union Carbide	Sumitomo Chemical, Daiichi Seiyaku, Mitsubishi Chemicals & Petrochemicals, Kyowa Hakko Kogyo, Toatsu Mitsui Chemicals, Asahi Chemical, Ajinomoto, Takeda Chemical, Daicel Chemical, Kirin Brewery, Hoshida Pharmaceutical, Nippon Kayaku, Nippon Oil, Oji Paper, Sanyo Chemical, Suntory, Shionogi, Green Cross	Rhone-Poulenc, Moet-Hennessy, Elf Aquitaine, BSN-Gervais-Danone, Air Liquide, Roussel-Uclaf, Lafarge Coppee	Grand Metropolitan (U.K.), Shell (U.K. & Neth.), B.P. (U.K.), IMCO (Can.), Hoffman - La Roche (Swiss), Kabi Vitrum (Sweden), Sandoz (Swiss), Ciba-Geigy (Swiss), Imperial Chemicals (U.K.), BASF (W. Ger.), Hoechst (W. Ger.)
Multi-Organization	Whitehead Inst. (MIT)	Bio-Technology Project (MITI)	Transgene, Societe Lyonnaise [Institut Pasteur]	Celltech (U.K.), NEB (U.K.)

FIGURE 11. Representative and partial list of institutions participating in the biotechnology industry.

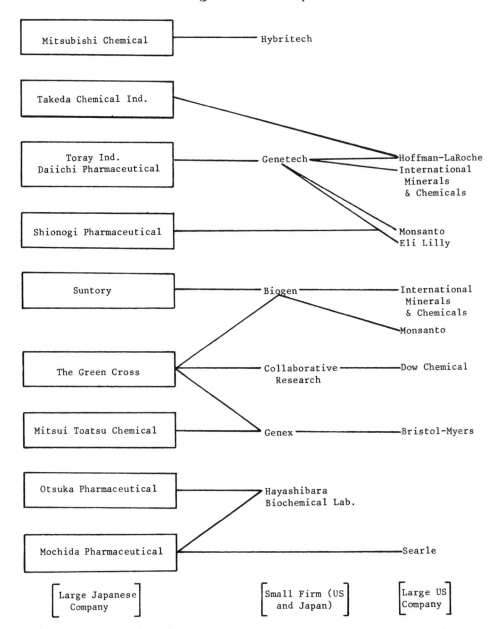

FIGURE 12. Relationships between US and Japanese biochemical companies.

We wanted to test, then, even against this bias, whether such companies were using and are going to continue to use a greater variety of technology strategy approaches and a greater proportion of external techniques for technology development than they had employed in the past.

Several methods for technology development and acquisition were identified (Table 3).[33] Technologies developed in the industrial R&D laboratory or in entrepreneurial subsidiaries represent the fruits of internal techniques of development.

TABLE 3. Technology development and acquisition approaches

Internal
    1. Technologies Developed Originally in the Central R&D Lab or Division
    2. Technologies Developed Using Internal Venturing, Entrepreneurial
       Subsidiaries, Independent Business Units, etc.

External
    3. Technologies Developed Through External Contracted Research
    4. External Acquisitions of Firms for Primarily Technology-Acquisition Purposes
    5. As A Licensee for Another Firm's Technology
    6. Joint Ventures to Develop Technology
    7. Equity Participation in Another Firm to Acquire or Monitor Technology
    8. Other Approaches for Technology Development or Acquisition

Source: Adapted from Edward B. Roberts, "New Ventures for Corporate Growth," *Harvard Business Review*, July–August, 1980.

The remaining techniques are considered to be the external methods of technology development or acquisition.

Ninety-seven companies met our R&D expenditure criterion, and are listed in Table 4.

Sixteen companies were selected to give a preliminary indication of the direction of our study results. The 97 companies fell within 24 industry groupings (*Business Week*'s classifications), while the subset of 16 fell within seven industry groupings (Table 5).

Data were gathered by three methods: 1) comparative analysis of *Wall Street Journal Index* citations; 2) analysis of annual reports and 10-Ks; and 3) phone interviews based on a common questionnaire.

The *Wall Street Journal Index* citations for the first 16 firms studied for the years 1978 and 1983 were scanned for any mention of a company's use of one of the techniques of technology acquisition or development. The years were chosen by taking the most recent year and the year five years previous to it.

The results of the *Index* search are listed in Table 6. There has obviously been both an increase in the general variety of use of approaches and a significant increase in the use of each individual method of external technology acquisition. Companies that have strong in-house research capabilities have been using, at the same time, more of and a greater variety of external sources.

To test whether the two years chosen for the study may not have just been anomalies, annual reports and phone interviews were used to corroborate or refute the direction of the findings. The annual reports were scanned for any mention of a company's use of one of the techniques. This information was used as a recall aid for the respondents. In-depth phone interviews were completed for ten of the 16 companies. In the phone interviews, respondents were asked questions about methods of technology-strategy planning and about trends over the past five to seven years and for the next five to seven years in the use of technology development techniques. The interviews required two or three respondents from each company and

TABLE 4. Companies that spent more than $80 million on R&D in 1982

Abbott	J&J
Allied	Lilly
Allis-Chalmers	Litton
Aluminum Company of America	Lockheed
Amdahl	Martin Marietta
American Cyanamid	McDonnell-Douglas
American Home Products	Merck
American Motors	Mobil
AMP	Monsanto
Atlantic Richfield	Motorola
ATT	National Semiconductor
Baxter Travenol	NCR
Boeing	Northrop
Bristol-Meyers	Pfizer
Burroughs	P&G
Caterpillar	Phillips Petroleum
Celanese	Polaroid
Chrysler	PPG
Control Data	Raytheon
Corning Glass	RCA
Data General	Revlon
Dart & Kraft	Rockwell
DEC	Rohm & Haas
Deere	Schering-Plough
Dow	Schlumberger
DuPont	Searle
Eastman Kodak	Shell
Eaton	Signal
Emerson	SmithKline
Exxon	Socal
FMC	Sperry
Ford Motor	Squibb
GE	Standard Oil (Ind.)
General Dynamics	Syntex
General Foods	Tektronix
General Motors	Texaco
Goodyear	Textron
Gould	3M
GTE	TI
Gulf	TRW
Halliburton	Union Carbide
Harris	United Technologies
Hewlett-Packard	Upjohn
Honeywell	U.S. Steel
IBM	Wang
Ingersoll-Rand	Warner-Lamber
Intel	Westinghouse
International Harvester	Xerox
ITT	

Source: *Business Week*, March 21, 1984

**TABLE 5. Listing of industry groups represented by companies
that spent more than $80 million on R&D in 1982**

Aerospace
Automotive: cars, trucks
Automotive: parts, equipment
*Chemicals
Conglomerates
*Drugs
Electrical
Electronics
Food & Beverage
Fuel
*Information Processing: Computers
Information Processing: Office Equipment
Instruments
*Leisure Time Industries
Machinery: farm & construction
Machinery: machine tools, industrial, mining
Metals & Mining
*Miscellaneous Manufacturing
Oil Service & Supply
*Personal & Home Care Products
Semiconductors
Steel
*Telecommunications
Tire & Rubber

*Industries from which companies were studied in further detail.
Source: *Business Week*, March 21, 1984

**TABLE 6. Technology development activity
of selected 16 firms, 1978 and 1983**

	(# of Publicly Reported Major Instances of Technology Strategy Activities)	
Approach	1978	1983
1. R&D Lab	—	1
2. Internal Venturing	0	4
3. Contracted Research	1	7
4. Acquisition of Firms	10	18
5. Licensee	5	9
6. Joint Venture	1	16
7. Equity Participation	0	8
8. Other (Market Another's Product)	5	14
Totals	21	77

Source: *Wall Street Journal Index*, 1978 & 1983.

took about an hour each to complete. (The questionnaire upon which the phone interviews were based is included as an appendix to this article.)

Respondents were asked to allocate the significance of the use of each technology development or technology acquisition activity within the corporation by using proportional measures. One hundred percent represented the entire set of such activities. The change in the proportion over the time period was used as the direction indicator in Table 7.

A negative sign, as in the use of the central R&D lab, for example, does not mean that the activity decreased on an absolute scale. For example, R&D funding was not necessarily cut. Rather, the *relative* importance of the central R&D lab decreased compared to the other technology development or acquisition activities.

The interview results corroborate the *Wall Street Journal Index* search in that the external sources of technology development grew in relative importance over the past few years at the expense of the central R&D lab. There was also a shift in relative importance internally from the central R&D lab to internal ventures or to entrepreneurial subsidiaries for R&D development. For the period that lasted from the late 1970s through the mid-1980s, press reports, annual reports, and the observations of corporate planners and R&D managers generally all indicate an increase in the variety of activities used for technology development and an increase in the relative importance of external sources over internal ones.

In the interviews, we also asked whether these trends were likely to continue in the future. We found different results (Table 8).

The recent and current period of experimentation, which has been characterized by the expansion of both external-oriented approaches and a greater variety generally of types of innovation efforts, may be stabilizing. Many of our respondents paint a near-term future of more consolidation in technology strategy methods. The central R&D lab is not generally predicted to lose any more relative significance, and it may stabilize at its present level of importance. Some of the other activities,

TABLE 7. Directional change in relative significance for the eight approaches for ten companies, 1978–1984

Approach	+	0	−
1. R&D Lab	0	5	5
2. Internal Venturing	4	6	0
3. Contracted Research	2	8	0
4. Acquisition of Firms	6	3	1
5. Licensee	4	5	1
6. Joint Venture	5	5	0
7. Equity Participation	3	6	1
8. Other (Market Another's Product)	3	7	0

+ increase in relative significance
0 no change in relative significance
− decrease in relative significance

Source: Personal Interviews

TABLE 8. Directional change in relative significance for the eight approaches for ten companies, 1984–1990

Approach	+	0	−
1. R&D Lab	0	8	2
2. Internal Venturing	2	6	2
3. Contracted Research	1	8	1
4. Acquisition of Firms	5	3	2
5. Licensee	5	4	1
6. Joint Venture	5	3	2
7. Equity Participation	2	6	2
8. Other (Market Another's Product)	2	7	1

+ increase in relative significance
0 no change in relative significance
− decrease in relative significance

Source: Personal Interviews

moreover, may lose relative priority. The broad range of external activities may be used somewhat less, although three activities may continue to grow in relative importance. These activities are the formation of joint ventures, licensing, and the buying of firms for technology acquisition and development.

In the interviews, respondents were also asked about the location in the organizational hierarchy of those people performing technology-strategy planning. Technology-strategy planning was defined as consisting of the following activities:

- Determining what new markets or distribution channels a company can enter with its present technical capabilities;
- Determining the allocation of R&D funding for present major product lines;
- Determining what new technologies to develop or acquire; and
- Determining the methods of technology acquisition or development.

TABLE 9. Location of technology-planning activity

Location \ Company	A	B	C	D	E	F*	G	H	I	J
HQ	X	X	X	X			X	X	X	X
Group	X		X	X						
Division				X	X					
SBU	X	X	X	X			X		X	X
Separate Technical Planning	X									
Lab	X		X	X						
Other										X

*Would not divulge information

Source: Personal Interviews

All the respondents who would discuss their firms' methodologies for technology-strategy planning said that their firms are explicitly performing this planning activity somewhere within the organization (Table 9).

Eight of the ten firms had people at corporate headquarters performing the function, and seven firms had people on two or more levels performing the function. Technology-strategy planning appears to be a multi-level and increasingly general management task.

Conclusion

As can be seen from our discussions and analyses at the historical and conceptual level, the industry level, and the firm level, technology appears to have evolved into a true strategic factor. In practically all types of technology-intensive industries—such as a fluid one like diagnostic ultrasound, one with a typical high-technology evolutionary cycle like personal computers, a revitalized formerly "sick" industry like machine tools, and a strategically managed one like biotechnology—strategic linkages and varied structures for encouraging innovation are increasingly crucial. Also, several corporations appear to have some form of headquarters involvement in technology-strategy planning. Moreover, technology strategy seems to be an increasingly diverse and multi-level activity.

Theoretically, there has always existed a number of approaches for developing or acquiring technology. These approaches can be segmented by development internally or acquisition and development externally. Within each segment, moreover, there exists some choice in the methods of development that are available. For internal development, a firm can use its own industrial R&D staff at the corporate level and within the divisions. A firm can also establish internal ventures or entrepreneurial units to develop technology. Externally, a firm can license technology or contract for its development, form a joint venture, or acquire part or all of another firm for monitoring or buying technology.

Even though these approaches have always existed, it appears that firms have just recently started to experiment seriously with a variety of these approaches. Our data show that firms have substantially increased their relative use of *all* techniques—other than using their own R&D staffs—for technology development. Along with increasing the use of a number of approaches, the firms have been relatively more active in employing the external approaches for development. These trends are corroborated by our analysis of four diverse technology-intensive industries.

There is also a general trend in technology strategy toward more cooperation among competitors for technology development, where firms use such methods as licensing, joint ventures, and acquisitions to share technology. This pattern may indicate that companies are using technology *per se* less and less as a purely competitive tool. As technology becomes more common, competition may shift away from technology and toward other areas, such as marketing and manufacturing.

A factor running counter to such an argument, however, is the prediction that the use of external sources as a group may level off. Intense experimentation of diverse technology strategy methods that stress cooperation may be unstable in the long run because of a lack of direct and full control, and because of the ultimate attraction of being fully and solely competitive for many corporations. If technology is to be used as a competitive weapon, one would predict less growth of cooperation among firms in sharing technology and a decreased growth rate in the use of several external-oriented approaches. According to this argument, therefore, the use of external-oriented methods may peak, and some consolidation may take place with a renewed focus on internal-oriented methods and on external-oriented efforts that are more directly under corporate management's control. The data tend to support this contention.

Technology, in summary, has become a strategic concern to all types of technology-intensive industries. A blending of previous technological innovation modes is taking place. Technology strategy is practiced by most technology-based companies in a multi-level manner. A period of rapid growth in the use of external-oriented strategic practices for technology acquisition has occurred over the past few years. Perhaps the more extensive use of external-oriented methods indicates greater cooperation within the industry, which, in turn, means that technology will be used less as a purely competitive tool. But the use of external-oriented approaches may be reaching an unstable state. Some consolidation back to the internal-oriented practices may be likely. As indicated in Figure 13, there appears to be a limit to intensive strategic diversity as large firms begin to attempt to reassert greater proprietary control over their technological resources.

It is clear that, starting in the middle or late 1970s, we have experienced a tremendous flurry of experimentation, creativity and variety in the area of technology strategy. The earlier and simpler situation, consisting primarily of separate spheres

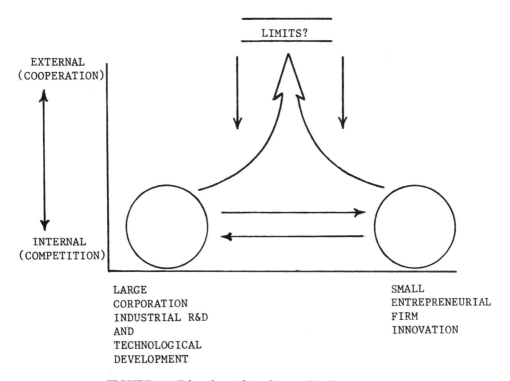

FIGURE 13. Direction of modern technology strategy.

of technological innovation in the private sector, is probably over. But there may also be limits to this exciting wave of managerial development. Complexity may be too great. The desire to internalize or to gain total proprietary control may strengthen. Perhaps, by the 1990s, a mini-backlash may develop. But even then, with some consolidation, technology strategy has emerged. It will remain more varied and complex than technological innovation was two decades ago, and technology will continue to be an essential part of strategic management.

Notes

1. For a discussion of the neglect of technology in the traditional strategic management literature, see Mel Horwitch, "The Blending of Two Paradigms for Private-Sector Technology Strategy" in Jerry Dermer, ed., *Competitiveness Through Technology: What Business Needs from Government* (Lexington, MA: Lexington Books, Inc., in press); and Alan Kantrow, "The Strategy-Technology Connection," *Harvard Business Review*, July–August 1980.

2. For the process of technological innovation, see Donald G. Marquis, "The Anatomy of Successful Innovations," *Innovation*, no. 7 (1969); *Success and Failure in Industrial Innovation: Report on Project Sappho* (London: Centre for the Study of Industrial Innovation, no date); R. Rothwell *et al.*, "SAPPHO Updated: Project SAPPHO Phase II," *Research Policy*, Vol. 3 (1974), pp. 258–291; James Utterback, "The Process of Technological Innovation Within the Firm," *Academy of Management Journal*, March 1971, pp. 75–88. For the technology-organization structure discussion, see J. Woodward, *Industrial Organization: Theory and Practice* (London: Oxford University Press, 1965); D. Hickson, D.S. Pugh and D. Pheysey, "Operations Technology and Organizational Structure: An Empirical Reappraisal," *Administrative Science Quarterly*, Vol. XIV (1969), pp. 378–396; G.G. Stanfield, "Technology and Organization Structure As Theoretical Categories," *Administrative Science Quarterly*, Vol. XXI (1976), pp. 489–493. For the role of technology in the international product life cycle, see Louis T. Wells, Jr., "International Trade: The Product Life Cycle Approach" in Louis T. Wells, Jr., ed., *The Product Life Cycle and International Trade* (Boston: Harvard Business School Division of Research, 1972), pp. 3–33.

3. For necessary interactions with the market and the user, see Donald G. Marquis, "The Anatomy of Successful Innovations"; *Success and Failure in Industrial Innovation: Report on Project Sappho*; R. Rothwell *et al.*, "SAPPHO Updated: Project SAPPHO Phase II"; Eric von Hippel, "The Dominant Role of Users in the Scientific Instrument Innovation Process," *Research Policy*, Vol. 5 (1976), pp. 212–239. For discussions about the need for champions, entrepreneurs and technology-familiar managers, see Donald A. Schon, "Champions for Radical New Inventions," *Harvard Business Review*, March–April 1963; Donald A. Schon, *Technology and Change* (New York: Delacorte, 1967); Edward B. Roberts, "Entrepreneurship and Technology," *Research Management*, July 1968; Edward B. Roberts, "Generating Effective Corporate Innovation," *Technology Review*, October–November 1977; Robert Hayes and William Abernathy, "Managing Our Way to Economic Decline," *Harvard Business Review*, July–August 1980.

4. For typical strategic planning views emphasizing present-past portfolios, see Boston Consulting Group, *Perspectives on Experience* (Boston: The Boston Consulting Group, 1967); R.V. Buzzell, B.T. Gale and R.G.M. Sultan, "Market Share — Key to Profitability," *Harvard Business Review* January–February 1975; P. Haspeslagh, "Portfolio Planning: Uses and Limits, *Harvard Business Review*, January–February 1982. For the external-oriented strategy literature that uses very different approaches, see Michael Porter, *Competitive Strategy* (New York: Free Press, 1980); R. Edward Freeman, *Strategic Management: A Stakeholder Approach* (Marshfield, MA: Pitman, 1984). For an emphasis on the need for strategy to be supported by internal structures, systems and processes, see Alfred D. Chandler, Jr., *Strategy and Structure* (Cambridge, MA: MIT Press, 1962); Jay Galbraith and Daniel A. Nathanson, *Strategic Implementation: The Role of Structure and Process* (St. Paul, MN: West Publishing, 1978). For implicit strategy, see Chester Barnard, *The Functions of Executive* (Cambridge, MA: Harvard University Press, paperback edition, 1968); Kenneth R. Andrews, *The Concept of Corporate Strategy* (Homewood, IL: Richard D. Irwin, 1980); Thomas Peters and Robert Waterman, *In Search of Excellence* (New York: Harper and Row, Inc., 1982); R. Edward Freeman, *Strategic Management: A Stakeholder Approach*; J. Brian Quinn, *Strategies for Change: Logical Incrementalism* (Homewood, IL: Richard D. Irwin, 1980). For an early discussion of the distinctive modes of technological innovation, see Mel Horwitch and C.K. Prahalad, "Managing Technological Innovation — Three Ideal Modes," *Sloan Management Review*, Winter 1976.

5. Mel Horwitch, *The Golden Age of Corporate Strategy: The Rise of Strategic Planning in the 1960s and 1970s*, MIT Sloan School Working Paper, 1985. For the reaction to strategic planning, see Robert Hayes and William

Abernathy, "Managing Our Way to Economic Decline"; "The Future Catches Up with a Strategic Planner," *Business Week*, June 17, 1983, p. 62.

6. For a review of the rise of the small high-technology firm, see Edward B. Roberts, "A Basic Study of Innovations," *Research Management*, July 1968; Roy Rothwell, "The Role of Small Firms in the Emergence of New Technologies," *Omega*, Vol. XII, no. 1 (1984), pp. 19–29; Nancy S. Dorfman, *Massachusetts' High Technology Boom in Perspective: An Investigation of Its Dimensions, Causes and of the Role of New Firms*, CPA 82-2 (Cambridge, MA: Center for Policy Alternatives, MIT, 1982); James M. Utterback, *Technology and Industrial Innovation in Sweden: A Study of New Technology-Based Firms*, CPA 82-06/A (Cambridge, MA: Center for Policy Alternatives, MIT, May 31, 1983); Paul Freiberger and Michael Swaine, *Fire in the Valley* (Berkeley, CA: Osborne-McGraw-Hill, 1984); Michael S. Malone, *The Big Score: The Billion Dollar Story of Silicon Valley* (Garden City, NY: Doubleday & Co., Inc., 1985); Roger Miller and Marcel Cote, "Growing the Next Silicon Valley," *Harvard Business Review*, July–August 1985. For the attraction of the small-firm approach for stimulating innovation in large corporations, see James Brian Quinn, "Managing Innovation: Controlled Chaos," *Harvard Business Review*, May–June 1985; Edward B. Roberts, "New Ventures for Corporate Growth, *Harvard Business Review*, July–August, 1980.

7. For a recent discussion of the increasing importance of technology in Japanese corporate and national industrial strategy, see "Special Report: Japan's Technology Agenda," *High Technology*, August 1985, pp. 21–67.

8. Kiyonori Sakakibara, *From Imitation to Innovation: The Very Large-Scale Integrated (VLSI) Semiconductor Project*, MIT Sloan School Working Paper 1490-83, October 1983.

9. For various warnings of the technological competitive threat that Japan posed to the US, see Ezra Vogel, *Japan As Number 1: Lessons for America* (Cambridge, MA: Harvard University Press, 1979); Robert B. Reich, "Making Industrial Policy," *Foreign Affairs*, Spring 1982, pp. 852–888; Ira Magaziner and Robert B. Reich, *Minding America's Business* (New York: Vintage paperback edition, 1983); *U.S. Industrial Competitiveness: A Comparison of Steel, Electronics and Automobiles* (Washington, DC: U.S. Office of Technology Assessment, July 1981); *Commercial Biotechnology: An International Analysis* (Washington, DC: U.S. Office of Technology Assessment, January 1984); *International Competition in Advanced Industrial Sectors: Trade and Development in the Semiconductor Industry*, A Study Prepared for the Use of the Joint Economic Committee of the U.S. Congress (Washington, DC: U.S. Government Printing Office, February 18, 1983).

10. For perhaps the earliest call for a strategic view of manufacturing, see Wickham Skinner, "Manufacturing— Missing Link in Corporate Strategy," *Harvard Business Review*, May–June 1969. For a historical review of manufacturing management in the U.S., see Wickham Skinner, "The Taming of the Lions: How Manufacturing Leadership Evolved," chapter 20 in Wickham Skinner, *Manufacturing: The Formidable Competitive Weapon* (New York: John Wiley & Sons, Inc., 1985). For modern examples of a strategic view of manufacturing and of parallel calls for a strategic view of technology, see Robert Hayes and William Abernathy, "Managing Our Way to Economic Decline"; William Abernathy, Kim Clark and Alan Kantrow, *Industrial Renaissance* (New York: Basic Books, Inc., 1983); Robert Hayes and Steven C. Wheelwright, *Restoring Our Competitive Edge: Competing Through Manufacturing* (New York: John Wiley & Sons, Inc., 1984); Charles H. Fine and Arnoldo C. Hax, "Manufacturing Strategy: A Methodology and an Illustration," *Interfaces*, Vol. 15, no. 6 (November–December 1985).

11. For the current trend in strategic management that emphasizes such concerns as corporate culture, implementation and global issues, see Thomas Peters and Robert Waterman, *In Search of Excellence*; Michael Porter, *Competitive Advantage* (New York: Free Press, 1985); Kenichi Ohmae, *Triad Power: The Coming Shape of Global Competition* (New York: Free Press, 1985); Arnoldo Hax and Nicoles Majluf, *Strategic Management: An Integrative Perspective* (Englewood Cliffs, NJ: Prentice-Hall, Inc., 1984); *Global Competition: The New Reality* (Washington, DC: The Report of the President's Commission on Industrial Competitiveness, Vol. II, January 1985).

12. For early calls for a strategic view and a broad synthesis of the management of technology field, see Richard S. Rosenbloom, "Technological Innovation in Firms and Industries: An Assessment of the State of the Art" in P. Kelly and M. Kranzberg, eds., *Technological Innovation: A Critical Review of Current Knowledge* (San Francisco: San Francisco Press, 1978); Richard S. Rosenbloom and William J. Abernathy, "The Climate for Innovation in Industry," *Research Policy*, Vol. 11 (1982), pp. 209–225.

13. Mel Horwitch and C.K. Prahalad, "Managing Technological Innovation—Three Ideal Modes"; Mel Horwitch, "The Blending of Two Paradigms for Private-Sector Technology Strategy."

14. See references in Note 6.

15. Christopher Freeman, *The Economics of Industrial Innovation* (Cambridge, MA: MIT Press, 1982), chapter 8.

16. For a more extensive discussion of the previous two separate modes for technological innovation and the current blending and blurring of them, see Mel Horwitch, "The Blending of Two Paradigms for Private-Sector Technology Strategy."

17. Mel Horwitch and Raymond A. Thiertart, *The Effect of Business Interdependencies on Technology-Intensive Business Performance: An Empirical Investigation*, MIT Sloan School Working Paper, 1658-85. July 2, 1985.

18. Information on the early history of the U.S. personal computer industry comes from the following sources: Paul Freiberger and Michael Swaine, *Fire in the Valley*; Gary N. Farner, *A Competitive Analysis of the Personal Computer Industry*, Sloan School of Management, MIT, unpublished master's thesis, May 1982; Deborah F. Schreiber, *The Strategic Evolution of the Personal Computer Industry*, Sloan School of Management, MIT, unpublished master's thesis, May 1983; Michael S. Malone, *The Big Score*; "A Microcomputing Timeline," *Byte*, September 1985, pp. 198–208; Mark Garetz, "Evolution of the Microprocessor," *Byte*, September 1985, pp. 209–215.

19. "Microcomputer Use Doubles in Past Year in Leading Organizations," Research and Planning, Inc., press release, circa June, 1984.

20. "Personal Computers and the Winner Is IBM," *Business Week*, October 3, 1983, pp. 76–95; Lawrence J. Curran and Richard S. Shuford, "IBM's Estridge," *Byte*, November 1983, pp. 88–97; Vrian Camenker, "The Making of the IBM PC," *Byte*, November 1983, pp. 254–256.

21. "IBM and Intel Link Up to Fend Off Japan," *Business Week*, January 10, 1983, pp. 96–97; *Wall Street Journal*, August 17, 1983, p. 10.

22. "AT&T Introduces Personal Computer," *New York Times*, June 17, 1984, p. D5; "AT&T's Long-Awaited Micro," *InfoWorld*, July 16, 1984, pp. 46–47.

23. "A Real Computer on Your Lap?," *InfoWorld*, April 2, 1984, p. 13.

24. *InfoWorld*, May 14, 1984.

25. For data and information on the medical equipment industry and the diagnostic ultrasound segment, see Derek Abell, *Defining the Business* (Englewood Cliffs, NJ: Prentice-Hall, Inc., 1980); Yves Doz and Richard Hamermesh, *Medical Products Group (A, B, C)* (Boston: HBS Case Services, 1975); *Medical Imaging Instruments* (New York: Frost & Sullivan, 1975); *Medical Ultrasound Imaging Equipment Markets in the U.S.* (New York: Frost & Sullivan, 1982); Betty Hamilton, ed., *Medical Diagnostic Imaging Systems* (New York: Frost & Sullivan, 1982); *The Medical Diagnostic Ultrasound Market* (New York: Klein Biomedical Consultants, 1980); *Electronics*, January 12, 1984; results of Diagnostic Ultrasound Industry Survey conducted by John Friar, May–September 1985.

26. For the key role of the machine tool industry in U.S. business history, see Nathan Rosenberg, "Technological Change in the Machine Tool Industry, 1840–1910," *Journal of Economic History*, Vol. XXIII, no. 4 (December 1963).

27. For a comprehensive industry analysis of the traditional U.S. machine tool industry, see National Research Council, *The U.S. Machine Tool Industry and the Defense Industrial Base* (Washington, DC: National Academy Press, 1983), chapter 2.

28. For robotics, see Mel Horwitch and Kiyonori Sakakibara, *The Changing Strategy-Technology Relationship in Technology-Related Industries: A Comparison of the United States and Japan*, Sloan School Working Paper, MIT, 1533-84, January 5, 1984.

29. For a general discussion of strategic groups, see Michael E. Porter, *Competitive Strategy*, chapter 7.

30. For the restructuring and broadening of the machine tool industry, see National Research Council, *The U.S. Machine Tool Industry and the Defense Industrial Base*, chapter 2.

31. See Mel Horwitch and Kiyonori Sakakibara, *The Changing Strategy-Technology Relationship*.

32. For a comprehensive discussion of the biotechnology industry, see Mel Horwitch and Kiyonori Sakikabara, *The Changing Strategy-Technology Relationship*.

33. Edward B. Roberts, "New Ventures for Corporate Growth."

Appendix
Technology Strategy Survey

This survey is part of a major study on the evolution and current state of technology strategy and technology planning in large corporations that compete in technology-intensive industries. We very much would like your participation. We have also tried very hard to keep this survey brief. Please feel free to make additional comments, elaborate on points, and include supplementary material that you think might relate to your answers or to the subject of the overall study. Of course, all company-specific answers that are not obviously available in the public domain will be kept confidential unless you release them. We will also share our findings with you. Thank you very much for your help.

John Friar
Mel Horwitch
MIT, Alfred P. Sloan School of Management
50 Memorial Drive, E52-556
Cambridge, MA 02139
Tel: 617-253-6672

I.   Name   _____

        Position   _____

        Company   _____

        Division,

        Subsidiary, etc. _____

        Address   _____

                        _____

                        _____

        Telephone   (   ) _____

        Today's Date   _____

II-1.   Could you please try to estimate how much of your company's overall business (in terms of percentage of sales) is technology-strategy/technology-planning relevant (i.e., in your opinion, uses or could use technology-strategy/technology-planning)?

II-2a-1. In terms of percentage of sales, how much of your current business is now covered by your technology-strategy or technology-planning process?

II-2a-2. Also, if it exists at all, where is explicit and/or formal technology strategy or technology planning practiced in your corporation?

        _____ Corporate Headquarters

        _____ The Group (i.e. Multi-Division) Level or Equivalent

        _____ The Division Level or Equivalent

        _____ The Business or Strategic Business Unit (SBU) Level or Equivalent

        _____ At the Central R&D Laboratory or Equivalent

        _____ At a Totally Separate Technology-Planning Unit or Equivalent (Please explain briefly if possible).

        _____ Elsewhere (Please explain briefly if possible).

II-2a-3. Also, if it is practical at all, we are interested in at least understanding in a general way *how* technology strategy or technology planning is practiced in your corporation. However, instead of answering an involved set of questions, could you possibly include some of the "raw" forms or other formal documents that are used or that describe your technology-strategy or technology-planning process? Thank you.

II-2a-4. Does your firm have integrative, inter-departmental units that have significant technology-strategy or technology-planning roles. If so, what is this unit(s) called, who heads it (position & name if possible), and when was it formed.

III.   We are also very interested in how your methods for technology development and technology acquisitions have evolved and will continue to evolve. We have listed below various methods and approaches for technology development and technology acquisition that are used by modern corporations. Beside each method there are three columns: the late 1970s; the mid-1980s (the present); and the early 1990s. We would like you to give us your best estimate for the entire range of technology-development and technology-acquisition activities practiced at your corporation for each of the three periods. Assuming that 100 percent represents the entire set of such activities, please estimate and allocate the approximate significance of each activity at your corporation using percentages for each period.

	Late 1970s	Mid-1980s (the present)	Early 1990s
1. Technologies Developed Originally in the Central R&D Lab.	____%	____%	____%
2. Technologies Developed Using Internal Venturing, Entrepreneurial Subsidiaries, Independent Business Units, etc.	____%	____%	____%
3. Technologies Developed Through External Contracted Research	____%	____%	____%
4. External Acquisitions of Firms for Primarily Technology-Acquisition Purposes	____%	____%	____%
5. As a Licensee for Another Firm's Technology	____%	____%	____%
6. Joint Ventures to Develop Technology	____%	____%	____%
7. Equity Participation in Another Firm to Acquire or Monitor Technology	____%	____%	____%
8. Other Approaches for Technology Development or Acquisition (Please Explain Briefly)	____%	____%	____%
Total	100%	100%	100%

IV-a.   For your most recent fiscal year, could you please list the specific technologies that have been commercially introduced, the specific joint ventures, equity positions or units established, and/or outside firms involved under each of the categories below.

1. Technologies Developed Originally in the Central R&D Lab.

2. Technologies Developed Using Internal Venturing, Entrepreneurial Subsidiaries, Independent Business Units, etc.
3. Technologies Developed Through External Contracted Research
4. External Acquisitions of Firms for Primarily Technology-Acquisition Purposes.
5. As a Licensee for Another Firm's Technology.
6. Joint Ventures to Develop Technology.
7. Equity Participation in Another Firm to Acquire or Monitor Technology.
8. Other Approaches for Technology Development or Acquisition (Please Explain Briefly).

IV-b. Specifically for your current joint ventures, could you please list your partners in the following matrix?

	Small Firms (under $50 million sales)	Large Firms (over $50 million in sales)
U.S. Firms		
Non-U.S. Firms		

IV-c. Specifically for your current equity participation positions, could you please list the firms in which you have equity interests in the following matrix?

	Small Firms (under $50 million sales)	Large Firms (over $50 million in sales)
U.S. Firms		
Non-U.S. Firms		

V. General data on your firm that is related to technology.
   a. In what industries do you compete?
   b. R&D spending as a percentage of total sales?
   c. R&D manpower as a percentage of total manpower?
   d. Annual number of patents issued?

Corporate Research and Development
The Latest Transformation
Margaret B.W. Graham

ABSTRACT. *This article assesses the implications for the conduct of corporate research of recent changes in industrial competition. It gives an evolutionary perspective on the strategic role of the corporate research laboratory, illustrating that role with examples from two major corporate research laboratories. It argues that, since 1975, a move toward greater diversity and experimentation in industrial R&D has posed complex and difficult operating problems for the corporate research laboratory as an institution, and that these problems need to be appreciated by those outside the research community if corporate research is to be an effective contributor to the formulation and execution of corporate strategy.*

Perhaps nowhere is the current international industrial realignment having more wrenching consequences than in the industrial research establishment. This article offers an evolutionary perspective on the state of the corporate research laboratory, the institution that has long symbolized industrial R&D in the United States. Historically, the corporate research laboratory has played an important role in shaping corporate strategy, one that has often been misunderstood by the nontechnical communities in corporations. Today corporations are acting to integrate technology with corporate strategic planning,[1] yet the strategic role of the corporate laboratory, what it is, and how it operates, remains a mystery to most managers and to almost all who practice or write about corporate strategic planning. This is particularly unfortunate, for it can lead to assignments for corporate laboratories which have infeasible — if not impossible — operating implications.

The role of corporate research in its institutionalized form has evolved through several distinct periods since the corporate research function originated at the turn of the present century.[2] The period before World War II saw the emergence of the corporate research center. It took place in a climate for industrial research that in-

Margaret B.W. Graham is Associate Professor of Operations Management at the Boston University School of Management. Dr. Graham holds an MBA from Harvard Business School and a Ph.D. in history from Harvard University. She has conducted research in the history and practice of industrial research and in the management of advanced manufacturing processes. In 1984–85 she was co-principal investigator on a National Science Foundation grant studying the Institutional Aspects of Procurement for Flexible Manufacturing Systems. Her work has been published in Decision Sciences, Harvard Business Review, *and in several reports published by the National Academy of Sciences. Her book, entitled* The Business of Research: RCA and the Videodisc, *is to be published by Cambridge University Press.*

volved little or no direct government funding of industrial R&D. Period Two, from 1941 to 1967, was the Age of Big Science, when government became directly involved in funding industrial R&D, and also encouraged competition between industrial R&D performers. The years 1967–1975 were a period of hiatus, a partial pullback when government gave up its dominant position in industrial R&D by deemphasizing R&D funding through defense.[3] The current era, beginning in 1975, presents us with yet another climate for industrial research. The intent of this paper is to explore the implications of the new climate for the context in which industrial research is performed, especially the implications that have bearing on the strategic role of the corporate laboratory.

Changes in the national climate for industrial R&D and in its corporate context have caused corporate laboratories to go through difficult transitional periods before. Such transitions have caused temporary but painful dislocations in their ability to participate in the formulation and execution of strategy. But the current dilemma of the corporate research laboratory as an institution may be more than a transitional problem. Created to meet focused objectives for corporate research in a much simpler national research environment, the typical corporate laboratory is facing a new and more complex mission. Many companies are experimenting with multiple new outside sources for technology, and are tapping them through mechanisms and relationships largely unknown to the previous research generation. The resulting hybrid approach to R&D could exacerbate the natural tension between R&D and the rest of the corporation: Clearly it poses difficult operational problems for the effective management of R&D institutions.

There is a growing body of historical research on industrial R&D, though until recently most of it stopped at World War II.[4] While this paper is informed by that research, it is based primarily on intensive historical and longitudinal studies at two of the 30 largest corporate laboratories in the United States, one at Alcoa, a major materials company, and the second at RCA, a diversified electronics company.[5] These laboratories, the first founded just after World War I, the second at the start of World War II, represent two important classes of industrial research laboratories, pursuing similar technology life-cycles at different periods of time. The first class includes such chemistry-based industries as chemicals, petroleum and metals, while the second class, including electronics, aeronautics and nuclear power, bases its technology on physics and chemistry.

Liferaft or White Elephant?

Why does the new industrial competition pose a threat to the corporate research center? The new industrial competition has shifted the international basis of competition toward technology at a time when much of American industry has either forfeited its previous technological edge or is struggling to maintain a tenuous lead.[6] Companies have tried to respond to low-cost, high-quality competition in two ways: by lowering their production costs and extending their existing product lines, and by bringing out new products and services at an ever-increasing rate. In short, they are trying simultaneously to increase the rapidity of incremental improvement in their existing businesses and to engage in technological leapfrogging to regain leading-edge positions. Both strategies require considerable degrees of technical support at a level of sophistication that in many large companies resides primarily in the corporate R&D center. These organizations, formerly often ignored as irrelevant by other parts of their companies, have been besieged with requests for support in developing new business opportunities and new processes, and for improving existing products and processes all at the same time.

Corporate R&D as Operations

The corporate R&D function is that part of R&D that falls directly under top management's purview. It concerns itself primarily with work that is judged to be of benefit to the corporation at large, rather than to individual pieces of it. Corporate research and development can encompass a wide variety of activities, but such activities can generally be grouped under two broad corporate strategic purposes. Table 1 depicts these two purposes for investing in corporate R&D activity, one motivated by relatively short-term technical needs that are in some sense generic to multiple parts of the corporation, the other motivated by the desire to insulate some R&D activity from day-to-day operating concerns and to focus it on long-term corporate needs outside the current scope of any operating divisions.[7] Many individual corporate R&D centers have alternated their focuses back and forth between these two purposes in the course of their evolution.

Table 2 suggests the type of structural and managerial arrangements that are generally associated with the two different corporate R&D missions.

TABLE 1. Alternative strategic purposes for corporate research

Long-Term — Opportunity Generating

> Build stock of usable technology
> Insulate researchers from day-to-day operating pressures
> Protect research budget from short-term fluctuations
> Set corporate-wide goals
> Nurture nascent businesses that may replace existing ones
> Encourage interdisciplinary stimulation
> Provide attractive high-class research environment

Short-Term — Generic Cost Reduction

> Apply on the shelf technologies to existing businesses
> Ration scarce specialist support needed by several divisions
> Spread cost of specialized facilities and people
> Avoid redundancy
> Transfer technology from outside sources or support purchase
> Transfer technology within corporation
> Maintain corporate-wide standards based on technical control
> Provide objective technological evaluation
> Mediate internal technical disputes

**TABLE 2. Managerial and structural approaches
to different R&D missions**

Long-Term — Opportunity Generating

    Discipline-based organization
    Openness to outside sources
    Laboratory control over research priorities
    Protection from daily operating contact
    Small group or individual researcher project size
    Theoretical, not experimental approach

Short-Term — Generic Cost Reduction

    Project Organization
    Close linkage with primary users
    Secrecy and little contact with outside world
    Large team project organization
    Experimental, rather than theoretical research approach
    End user decides research priorities

The corporate R&D organization, whether laboratory or integrated technical center, has always been something of an anomaly in corporate life. To quote Lowell Steele, ". . . it is possible for a function such as research and development to cease to be new, even to be used extensively by a corporation, and still fail to qualify as a member of the business team."[8] Whatever the strategic purpose of their work at a particular time, R&D personnel have tended to be different from other operating personnel. Although only a small proportion of the work that is performed by the average corporate R&D center has ever been fundamental work, much of it has been exploratory. Highly uncertain by nature, it has often required researchers to devote decades of their lives to research that would never see the light of day in any form, published or embodied. People who deal with so much ambiguity in their work often need security and stability in their surroundings. Consequently corporate R&D has combined needs for secure employment and stable funding with a highly unpredictable but generally lumpy pattern of output. Such an irregular flow of work, so unlike the ideal constant flow of other operating environments, has made the R&D organization especially vulnerable to criticism and resentment from other parts of the organization and to fluctuations in funding and other forms of support.

Research personnel have also been set apart by their professional status. Scientific researchers and research engineers have typically served two masters; while loyal to the companies that have employed them, they have also been influenced in their research priorities by the professions that have judged the quality of their work and rewarded their efforts. To manage a corporate laboratory, therefore, has been to perform a difficult balancing act in which the special needs of a particular corporation have had to be weighed against the sometimes countervailing forces at work in the national research climate. The strategic role of a particular corporate research organization at any given time has thus been determined by three things: the state of its core technology, its corporate context, and the prevailing climate for research at the national level.

Climatic Evolution

The national climate for industrial research in any particular era has depended upon such factors as the current relationship between different research-performing institutions, the pattern of research funding, the supply of trained researchers, and the prevailing philosophy concerning the proper role of research. In all of the three eras set forth earlier, these factors have been different. Here we will focus mainly on the post-World War II era, which superficially seems most similar to the current era in its heavy emphasis on R&D and the importance of technology.

This post-war era, which we have called the Age of Big Science, was the first time that the shape of R&D in industry began to be influenced by government funding. Funding patterns recorded by the National Science Foundation for the years between 1945 and 1966 tell the story. Total expenditures for R&D in the United States rose from $1.5 billion in 1945 to nearly $20 billion in 1966. Between 1953 and 1963 the amount of the total funded by the Federal Government, but performed by industry, increased from $1.4 billion to $7.3 billion. In the same single decade, basic research performed by industry increased from $151 million in 1953 to $522 million in 1963.[9]

After World War II, the government and all research performers — universities, government laboratories, and industrial laboratories — were committed to making the United States scientifically self-sufficient as a way of ensuring that the country would not again be dependent upon other countries for science as it had been on English and German scientists during and after World War II.[10] Two key changes resulted from the commitment to fund research as a national priority. For the first time in peacetime, government provided a major share of the money for industrial R&D, rising from 40% in the 1950s to 60% in the 1960s.[11] Government pursued a policy of increasing the number of companies that were serious research performers. As a consequence, during the 1950s, industrial research became a competitive business. Companies like RCA and Alcoa which had been unchallenged technology leaders were no longer the sole research performers in their industry, and other research-performing institutions joined the competition. Whereas industry had previously left fundamental or generic research to academia, during the 1950s each began to invade the other's research territory.

Although basic research never accounted for more than 10% of the total of R&D funding, it had a critical influence on the values of the industrial research community at large. Two particularly powerful influences were an emphasis on "technology push" (the view of technological innovation as a unidirectional transfer of knowledge from basic science through development and commercialization), and the belief in breakthrough innovations often leading to entirely new industries and blockbuster businesses (*e.g.*, the transistor or nylon). These views of the innovation process were reflected both in the way industry structured its technical resources and in the way the Federal Government distributed its funding.

Federal R&D funding in the post-war Age of Big Science focused heavily on two industries that became synonymous in their day with "high tech." These were electronics and aeronautics — fields in the early stages of the technology life-cycle, heavily dependent upon the scientific discipline of physics for their knowledge base, seemingly the most applicable to weapons systems, and apparently still possessing the possibility of fundamental breakthroughs for advancing the stock of available knowledge. By contrast, older research-performing industries, such as chemicals, petroleum, or aluminum, which had built their fundamental stock of technology in the interwar years, moved toward an emphasis on applications, most often approaching it through a less dramatic but more predictable incremental innovation process.

In the post-war era, sizeable increases occurred in other areas of industrial research, but these were funded to a much greater extent by the companies themselves.[12] Over all, the demand for research personnel increased dramatically, but the supply did not. When total funding for R&D increased 14 times between 1943 and 1963, for instance, the number of research scientists and research engineers increased four times. As a consequence, salaries of all technical personnel grew considerably, while salaries of scarce personnel, such as Ph.D. physicists, increased out of proportion to other specialties.[13]

The Age of Big Science might have run its course in a decade had not the Cold War and the Space Program elevated science to a national obsession.[14] After Sputnik, the strain on scarce research resources pushed up the price of industrial research. It came to an end in the 1970s: A sharp cutback in government funding of industrial R&D occurred because policy-makers lost faith in the idea that R&D was one of the levers by which government could promote technological innovation and productivity.[15]

Table 3 summarizes the chief characteristics of the climate for industrial research in the Age of Big Science. Chief among them were the belief in basic research and in technology-push, resulting in blockbuster innovations based on science, the new research-performing partnership between government and industry, coupled with sharp rivalry among research performers, and the mission directed at national scientific self-sufficiency.

Contextual Evolution: The RCA and Alcoa Examples

The context for industrial research has typically been a function of (1) the way a corporation's technical resources are organized; (2) the character of the institutions that perform its R&D; and (3) the mechanisms by which R&D is translated into commercial value. In many corporations, especially those in the focal industries for federal funding of R&D, these factors changed dramatically during the post-war era. Although few corporate R&D efforts could have been said to be formally inte-

---

TABLE 3. Post-World War II climate for industrial research

Philosophy of Basic Research Primacy
Commitment to National Self-Sufficiency in Research
Belief in Blockbuster Innovations
Federal Funding for Industrial R&D
Defense Channels for R&D Funding to Focal Industries
Models of Unidirectional Flow and Technology Push
Competition between Research Performers

TABLE 4. Post-World War II context for industrial research

Divisional Status for Corporate Research
Movement towards Consolidation of R&D
Remote Locations for R&D Facilities
Campus-like Environments for R&D
Secrecy and Insularity
Competition for Scarce Research Personnel
Entrepreneurial Role for Corporate Laboratories

grated into strategic planning in the 1950s and 1960s, the relationship between R&D and the rest of the corporation changed substantially.

Table 4 summarizes the key contextual trends that characterized corporate R&D after World War II. During this period, many large companies that did not already have corporate laboratories established such units. Moreover, several firms with industrial research laboratories gave them separate divisional status during this time. It became commonplace for large companies to operate corporate research divisions staffed by a high proportion of Ph.D.s, removed from operating locations and modeled on university campuses.

While part of the rationale for creating these remote research sites had to do with maintaining tight security for the increasingly large component of defense-related research, another factor was the need to compete for scarce research manpower. High salaries and pleasant surroundings were required to attract the best people among a group much in demand by the increased number of research-performing companies. The required degree of secrecy and remoteness, the relative independence of R&D from corporate operating divisions for financial support, and the absence of linkage between the research staff and operating personnel in divisions eventually posed serious long-term barriers to communication. By the 1960s, the laboratory was seen to be irrelevant to the central concerns of the mainstream of the corporation. The effect of these changes in some technology-based companies was to make it increasingly difficult to transfer, and, therefore, to gain commercial benefit from technologies developed in corporate laboratories.

Corporate research divisions that reported directly to top management were obviously created for strategic purposes, but they functioned differently depending upon the particular purpose required. In some firms they were separated out and given very long-term missions, while in other firms existing corporate R&D organizations were consolidated with other types of technical support to make the total R&D effort more accessible and more responsive to the operating organizations.

The two different structural approaches to R&D were exemplified in RCA and Alcoa, respectively. Alcoa and RCA both restructured their R&D organizations in the post-war period. Each company fashioned its approach to R&D in response to the state of development of its particular core technology, but each also was affected in several ways by the changes we have noted in the industrial research climate. As a company in a focal industry, RCA was more directly influenced by the climatic changes, but both were affected by prevailing attitudes about innovation to the extent that each attempted to achieve at least one science-based "blockbuster" innovation. In neither company were these projects ultimately to achieve commercial success.

Alcoa

Alcoa had had a corporate research program since World War I, one of a diverse set of R&D-performing facilities located at various company production sites. In the 1920s and 1930s, the purpose of corporate R&D at Alcoa was long term to build the knowledge base for the entire aluminum industry, and the company employed some of the leading metallurgical researchers in the world, both at its Cleveland Laboratory and at its corporate research laboratory at New Kensington, Pennsylvania. Their work on basic aluminum technology formed the knowledge base for industrial and academic metallurgists alike.

In 1946, as a result of an unfavorable antitrust suit, Alcoa lost its virtual monopoly of primary aluminum production. Gradually during the course of the next two decades, most of Alcoa's R&D facilities consolidated on one rural site, 25 miles from corporate headquarters in Pittsburgh. R&D restructured itself to support Alcoa's new strategy. Not wanting its research into the fundamentals of aluminum to benefit all competitors in the industry, the R&D organization refocused its efforts toward applying its already large stock of knowledge. Alcoa's technical staff reduced its contact with the outside world, and adopted strict conventions of secrecy to protect its technical lead.

To achieve the necessary linkage with other parts of the corporation, Alcoa formed an active subcommittee system that gave end-users the opportunity to direct research priorities and allocate funding among projects. In this way, much of the Alcoa R&D program became closely tied in to operating efforts. The exception was one long-term project, the Alcoa Smelting Process, a wholly new technology designed to replace the conventional Hall-Heroult process employed by the entire industry. It was of such enormous competitive significance that it was known only to the team working on it and top management.

Begun in the 1960s, the Alcoa Smelting Process (ASP) was potentially disruptive to four or five of Alcoa's existing production sites. It reached the pilot phase in the late 1970s after 15 years of sustained effort. By the time the project could have come to the attention of planners, all of the key decisions concerning the technology and many of the decisions concerning its commercialization had been made at the laboratories.

According to the head of Alcoa's Technical Center, during the most intensive period of work on ASP, the project suffered from several problems: deficiencies in the stock of knowledge Alcoa had to draw upon, excessive secrecy, and time pressure.[16] The conditions under which the project developed precluded tapping outside sources of technology that might have compensated for the company's internal lack of expertise in some areas. All of these conditions were eminently suited to the incremental improvements to existing process technologies that were the main purposes of Alcoa's technical effort after the war, but they were operationally dysfunctional for the achievement of ASP's more radical goals.

RCA

RCA lost a different kind of technical monopoly in the decade after the war, but it too had to shift its strategy as a result of the government's insistence upon creating more competition in technology-based industries. In 1958, RCA was forced to relinquish its practice of domestic package licensing of over 5,000 radio-related patents, a change that substantially affected its ability to capture the benefits of leading-edge research.

RCA's corporate research laboratory, a merger of several former manufacturing laboratories, opened in 1941 on a remote rural site near the small university town of Princeton, New Jersey. The research center was charged at its inception with conducting top-secret defense R&D into such areas as radar and vacuum tubes. The laboratories became a separate research division, reporting to a senior officer in charge of Research and Engineering. As a leading electronics and radio communications company, RCA had been the fourth largest recipient of contract R&D funds from the Office of Scientific Research and Development during the war. After the war, it found itself in one of the focal areas singled out for heavy government funding of R&D.

Immediately after World War II, RCA's laboratory worked intensely on several new business opportunities for RCA's existing consumer electronics business, but from 1954 on it devoted itself to the long-term task of building the knowledge base in electronics. Any work on new products for the traditional businesses was left to RCA's new advanced development facilities in the various product divisions. Although these facilities received part of their funding from corporate R&D, they suffered constant fluctuations in other funding and raids on their engineering resources by the divisions. They also suffered from a sense of inferiority in comparison with the laboratories, and gradually became resentful and suspicious of them.

In the 1950s and early 1960s, corporate R&D at RCA was assigned the mission of staying at the forefront of all electronics research. As the field of electronics grew, this became an insurmountable task. The corporate research center was also expected to produce the new businesses that would keep RCA growing steadily, despite its membership in the highly volatile and cyclical electronics industry. The technical staff at the laboratories was comprised of a growing proportion of young Ph.D.s in science and engineering. The younger generation members of the technical staff generally possessed no commercial experience of any kind. Their work was regarded as exotic and irrelevant by most of the division managers who ran RCA's traditional businesses, although it produced follow-on business in the new government electronics and aerospace industries. The government-funded portion of RCA's R&D budget grew steadily into the 1960s, eventually accounting for well above 30% of the budget. The high level of government support had a price, for it required a specialized staff to handle the reporting and the record-keeping. Moreover, defense-related research, which generally imposed unique research priorities and lower economic standards of achievement on researchers, coordinated poorly with research directed at commercial objectives. On the other hand, outside sources of money — not under control of any RCA operating division — gave the laboratories' personnel the opportunity to pursue the questions of greatest interest to them professionally.

The single most important long-term research project that RCA conducted during the 1960s and 1970s was the RCA Videodisc project, which drew, in part, on the exploratory work first conducted under defense auspices. Research for the project began in the mid-1960s when it became clear that the cost of R&D was outrunning increases in government R&D funding. Foreseeing a time when they would have to depend upon divisional support again to maintain the stable budgets they needed, the laboratories' management promoted videoplayers as the ultimate new business opportunity for the consumer electronics industry.

The videoplayer research that eventually resulted in the Videodisc project involved a corporate commitment to a major new consumer entertainment systems business, designed to result in new manufacturing lines for several of the company's largest commercial divisions. Mindful of earlier problems with the high cost of color television and anxious to shift the priorities of researchers who had done primarily non-commercial work, the RCA laboratories' management emphasized for its videoplayer research projects rigid economic goals, rather than high performance goals. This led to a choice of a technological alternative, the capacitance approach, that was lower in cost, but also restrictive in its ability to support a range of performance options. General consultation that took place in the divisions about the product concept showed that the divisions thought performance features were more important than the laboratories did, but the laboratories insisted on retaining control over all technical decisions. Later, as RCA's competitors announced higher performance videoplayer alternatives, the project had to keep increasing its performance targets and pushing its technology to match the moving targets.

Meanwhile, the RCA Consumer Electronics Division, which had never supported the laboratories' choice of technology, pursued competing alternatives. In 1976, the Consumer Electronics Division, having lost the internal fight over technological alternatives, decided to market a Japanese-produced videocassette recorder that proved to be a direct competitor of the internally developed Videodisc.

By the time Videodisc was approaching market readiness in 1980, RCA's strategy had shifted away from its late 1950s emphasis on technological leadership in electronics to a rigorous high-volume, cost-cutting approach. Much of the laboratories' program was devoted to the supporting effort, but it continued to push for substantial investment in Videodisc R&D. In 1981, RCA's chairman — no risk-taker — found himself obliged to commit RCA to the highly risky venture of introducing Videodisc to the market. RCA needed a significant technology-based opportunity to restore a faltering consumer electronics business and to recapture its reputation for technological leadership. Only one internally generated option was available, the one that the laboratories had been harboring for so many years. Videodisc was withdrawn three years after its introduction, having lost out primarily to the Japanese version of the videocassette recorder that its own Consumer Electronics Division had successfully marketed.

Corporate R&D in Strategy

Recently several authors have pointed to the need to look more closely at the way R&D affects strategy formulation and execution. Together they have called into question assumptions that are often made by economists and policy-makers dealing with aggregate statistics: that strategy is formulated solely in a top-down manner; that long-range R&D can be formally planned.[18] In fact, R&D has had an effect on strategy formulation in two ways, formal and informal, and the more long-term its orientation has been, the less formal has been its involvement with strategy formulation.[19] Historically, corporate laboratories have often resorted to a form of internal entrepreneurship to circumvent the opposition of existing divisions and to push the more radical technologies they have developed into commercialization. They have been in a position to champion technologies leading to businesses of their own choosing, because of their influence with top management, because of their ability to find outside support for their research activities, because of their ability to protect long-term projects from close scrutiny, and because — when new opportunities have been needed — their options have been the only ones available on short notice.

Formal planning techniques, limited as they generally have been to five-year time horizons, have rarely had a formative influence on long-term R&D projects, whether process- or product-oriented, because, as economic entities, the projects have become visible quite late in their development cycles.[20]

Although the contexts for R&D at Alcoa and RCA were quite different in the post-war period — Alcoa's structured for short term, incremental innovation and application of existing knowledge in a fairly mature technology, and RCA's for building its knowledge base in the youthful field of electronics — both companies attempted the type of radical innovation that typified the prevailing innovation philosophy of the era. Begun in one research era and completed in another, both projects survived transitions in climate and context, but both also illustrated two facts of R&D life: the power of corporate laboratories to impose strategy on the rest of the organization, and the problems of mixing two different R&D approaches.

The problem both corporate laboratories encountered was that, while they could influence actual strategy formulation through informal but effective channels, they encountered heavy opposition at the execution stage. The operating tasks required to develop and commercialize major innovations were quite different from the tasks involved in other forms of corporate R&D activity, and the methods and priorities that were appropriate for their other activities proved dysfunctional for their radical innovations.

Moreover, in both companies, the existing operating divisions were stimulated to improve their alternative technologies, rather than to adopt the more radical ones backed by the laboratories. In effect, the corporate laboratories were forced to assume the role of corporate entrepreneur, but their ability to push for successful execution was undermined by the lack of commitment by other parts of the company.

The 1980s: R&D Diversity and New Hybrid Purpose

A look at the climate and context of industrial R&D in the 1980s reveals some major differences from the climate and context of the Age of Big Science. Table 5 summarizes these changes. After a decade-long hiatus (1966–1975), during which R&D budgets flattened out altogether, investment in industrial R&D has resumed a steady upward course with increases in industrial funding for the first five years of

TABLE 5. New era for industrial research: climate and context

New Climate
Primacy of Applications
Need to Leapfrog Scientifically
Federal R&D Funding Concentrated in Defense Channels
Encouragement for Cooperation

New Context
Emphasis on Applications and Transfer Internally
External Sources for Research and Development
Cooperative Research and Development
Multiple Options for Technology
Persistence of Unidirectional Model
Pressure on R&D Overhead
Hybrid Mission for Corporate Research

the 1980s averaging 14% per year. Although government R&D funding is once again increasing substantially, industrial funding for industrial R&D now contributes over 50%, and the proportion is much greater outside the defense-related industries. Government funding for R&D is once again highly concentrated in defense-related technologies.

While the funding scenario may look like a return to the Age of Big Science, in other respects the current era for industrial research promises to be quite different. This time government's emphasis is not on basic research and research self-sufficiency, but on applications and on dissemination of knowledge. Federal support for engineering was one of only two fields to receive funding that exceeded the rate of inflation between 1972 and 1982, and in 1982 it reported twice the concentration of funds reported a decade earlier.

Government influence through agencies and through legislation is now directed toward encouraging cooperation in R&D and transfer between sectors, industries and companies, trying to avoid the perceived problems of research competition that emerged in the last R&D upsurge.[21] At the same time, heavy government funding is directed toward fundamental research in a few key areas, chief among them artificial intelligence. Almost all non-defense-related R&D funding from the government has leveled off or been cut back. Only advanced computer science has received significant increases, averaging 12% per year in the early 1980s. Industry may be filling the funding gap for fundamental R&D performed in universities. Industrial funding for R&D research was the fastest growing source of R&D support, averaging 16% per year between 1972 and 1982.[22]

Recent studies of "new" approaches to innovation in large corporations point to changes in the context for research in response to the climatic shift outlined earlier. Most of the approaches involve ways of obtaining technology from parties outside the firm, alternatives to internal R&D. Far from being new, they were the only ways to acquire new technology before R&D became an internal corporate function for so many companies after World War II. They include contracted research from other firms or from university or independent research laboratories; acquisition of or equity participation in other firms with more advanced or complementary technologies; licensing and cross-licensing; joint ventures—either with competitors or with suppliers—in which technology is a shared activity. Since 1978, several long-term collaborative programs have been set up between universities and companies, including Harvard/Monsanto and MIT/Exxon. No one can say for sure what the real extent of cooperative research is, or how long it may last. A recent report of the National Science Board has questioned whether the upswing in research working agreements is a "permanent jump to a new level of interaction, or whether it is part of a cyclical upswing" caused by temporary shortages of research personnel and the need of universities to adjust to declining government support.[23]

All of the approaches mentioned have been in use by one company or another for decades.[24] The difference now is that many more companies seem to be experimenting with various outside sources of technology, placing relatively more emphasis on outside sources compared to inside sources, and using a combination of several approaches at the same time. Furthermore, because of the shift in government policy away from a hard-line approach to antitrust, more open cooperation between competitors or potential competitors is possible. Of 10 companies surveyed in three technology-intensive industries by one study, all reported a relative decrease in the importance of their R&D laboratories and a relative increase in the use of several outside sources of technology.[25]

While the shift toward cooperation and the use of multiple sources offers promise of improved access to ideas in industry, it also poses some problems for corporate R&D, in particular, that should be recognized. First, tapping multiple sources of research and development and engaging in cooperative efforts with different outside parties—whether competitors, advanced suppliers or universities—introduces a degree of complexity into R&D operations that makes the earlier problems of coping with strategic transitions or simultaneous radical and incremental innovations based on internal R&D pale by comparison. The motivation for companies to use outside sources can be a pragmatic recognition of temporary internal limitations or the choice not to cover certain technologies internally, but it can also be a mistaken view that tapping outside sources is less expensive. Companies that expect outside sources to serve as less expensive substitutes for inside investment in necessary technological support and that eliminate in-house technical staff rather than modifying the structure and skill-mix of in-house technical resources can find themselves in very difficult positions.

To acquire technology from outside sources requires new and diverse skills that range from higher-level gatekeeping to project management. It necessitates the ability to adapt technologies that have been developed only to a very generic level or—more difficult—to readapt technologies that have been developed in another very different institutional context. In companies that have been accustomed to employing mainly in-house research, too few members of corporate R&D organizations come equipped with such skills, and most operating divisions are understaffed in technical support functions that can handle advanced or highly specialized technologies. Authors Cohen and Mowery have made this point another way. Speaking of the problem of limited appropriability of the results of in-house R&D, they warn that "while limited appropriability may well contribute to insufficient R&D activity, limited transferability of R&D outputs may undermine firms' capacities to absorb fully the output of cooperative R&D efforts. . . . Cooperative research functions most effectively as a complement to, rather than a substitute for, the in-house research activities of firms." They emphasize that a firm must possess some level of firm-specific expertise to absorb the fruits of externally conducted R&D.[26]

One reason that corporations may underestimate the support requirements for using outside sources of technology is that the "technology push" notion of how technology-based innovation occurs has lingered on from previous research generations. The view that innovation originates neatly at one source and flows as water to passive receivers may be recognized as a gross distortion of reality, but it continues to be imbedded in the structures and policies of many companies. As the pressure to acquire, transfer and apply technology more speedily becomes greater, many companies place the responsibility for innovation and transfer firmly on the corporate R&D organizations without altering the incentives toward such behavior in the operating organizations. In time, corporate R&D may be blamed because it has been unable unilaterally to achieve a task that it ought never have been expected to accomplish without expert cooperation in the user organizations. Just as firms need complementary in-house skills to make use of research generated externally, so plants and other operating sites require a firm technology base to apply technology on site, to identify promising areas for potential process improvement, and to formulate research and development questions that can best be answered centrally.

A second type of change taking place in the corporate context for R&D in the current era is the use of more specialized organizations to accomplish different types of innovation. In particular, many companies are setting up formal venturing organizations,[27] and organizations charged with the task of transferring technology between operating divisions and from R&D to operations. Again, such structures are not really new; their use is becoming more widespread. Often they are established to avoid the pitfalls companies like Alcoa and RCA have encountered with their long-term, technology-based innovations in a previous era. And, again, unless they perform their own R&D, leading to a proliferation of unrelated and uncoordinated research efforts, such structures can increase still further the complex task of a corporate R&D organization.[28]

Surveying the current experimentation with multiple avenues for innovation, it is clear that, if R&D is to be "integrated" into corporate strategy at a time of increasing diversity, changes have to be made not only in the structure of the R&D function, but in the rest of the organization. To be sure, R&D needs to be taken into account in the strategy formulation process, but the operating implications of following different approaches to innovation must also be investigated and understood. To take full advantage of the "new" sources of technology, changes have to be made not only within the R&D organizations themselves, but also within the operating divisions. The all-too-common effort to reduce overhead by cutting costs at either end of this relationship is to render the entire investment meaningless. Neither abolishing the corporate R&D center and resorting to external alternatives nor changing the management approach, structure, funding or staffing of the corporate R&D organization will be sufficient, if the needs for complementary changes in the operating divisions are neglected.

Conclusion

Historically, corporate R&D centers have been dynamic organizations; they have survived and adapted to several major changes in the climate for industrial R&D, as well as changes in their own company strategies. Like all other organizational forms, they have had their limitations. The nature of their workforce has made it especially hard for them to change quickly. Moreover, they have performed poorly when required to handle several different approaches to R&D at the same time in the same organization. For this reason, the most difficult challenges managerially have occurred during transitional periods, when the old approach to R&D has proved to be inappropriate to the new mission. Long-term projects, those that have lasted for a decade or more in length, have been particularly susceptible to this kind of problem, as the cases of the ASP and Videodisc both demonstrate. In effect, both of these projects illustrate the serious difficulties of managing a hybrid R&D approach. They also illustrate the strategic influence of corporate R&D, so hard to harness by formal planning techniques, because the timing is so unpredictable and out of phase with normal planning horizons. Although R&D organizations have been part of the corporate structure for many years, they remain foreign bodies, used, but never accepted as part of the corporate team.

More than 10 years ago, Lowell Steele predicted that US industry would soon be required to adopt a mixed strategy for R&D, leading selectively, while relying on external technologies in other areas. This mixed strategy would be difficult and threatening, because companies, having tended formerly to structure themselves for one or the other approach, would have to accommodate themselves to both. It might, in fact, require that "on a much smaller scale we repeat the historical sequence that R&D has gone through."[29] Steele's prediction now seems to be coming true, as companies come to terms with the new industrial competition.

Corporate R&D organizations are being required to take on full responsibility for a hybrid function with inadequate and inappropriate resources to accomplish that function and with very little understanding of the challenges they face. If managers outside R&D recognize that corporate R&D organizations are currently having to adjust to a mix of approaches that would formerly have been regarded as incompatible within the same organization, they may be given time to adjust. Whether or not corporate R&D organizations continue to generate long-term research in-house, the ability to translate research performed elsewhere into usable technology for a specific firm will almost certainly remain a responsibility internal to the firm. For this purpose, if corporate R&D did not exist in some form, sooner or later it would have to be invented.

Perhaps the heart of the problem lies elsewhere, however, in the ability of new and existing operating organizations to take responsibility for building their own internal technology base, not as a substitute for, but as a counterpart to the resources at the corporate level. Without the willingness to treat R&D as a continuing day-to-day responsibility of every operating division, new sources of R&D are likely to prove even less effective than old ones. This may be the hidden implication of the often used but seldom understood phrase, "integrating R&D into corporate strategy."

Notes

1. Barry Bozeman, Michael Crow and Albert Link, *Strategic Management of Industrial R&D* (Lexington, MA: Lexington Books, 1984). In their chapter entitled "Involvement of R&D in Corporate Strategic Planning: Effects on Selected R&D Management Practices," Alden S. Bean, Norman R. Baker *et al.* quote Richard N. Foster as saying that technology needs to be the driving force in strategy formation in the 1980s if the United States is to be competitive in the international marketplace (p. 83). See also Edward Weil and Robert R. Cangemi, "Linking Long-term Research to Strategic Planning," *Research Management*, May–June 1983, pp. 32–39.
2. See Margaret B.W. Graham, "Industrial Research in the Age of Big Science" in Richard S. Rosenbloom, ed., *Research on Technological Innovation, Management and Policy*, vol. 2 (New York: JAI Press, 1985), pp. 47–79.
3. For a thorough discussion of past federal R&D policy from an economist's perspective, see R.R. Nelson, ed., *Government and Technical Change: A Cross-Industry Analysis* (New York: Pergamon Press, 1982), summarized in Richard R. Nelson and Richard N. Langlois, "Industrial Innovation Policy: Lessons from American History," *Science*, vol. 219 (February 18, 1983), pp. 814–819.
4. See Stuart W. Leslie, "Charles F. Kettering and the Copper-cooled Engine," *Technology and Culture* (1981); David C. Mowery, "Firm Structure, Government Policy, and the Organization of Industrial Research: Great Britain and the United States, 1900–1950, *Business History Review*, vol. 58 (Winter 1984); David S. Noble, *America by Design* (New York: Knopf, 1977); Leonard S. Reich, "Industrial Research and the Pursuit of Corporate Security: The Early Years of G.E. Labs," *Business History Review* (1980); George David Smith, *The Anatomy of a Business Strategy: Bell, Western Electric, and the Origins of the American Telephone Industry* (Baltimore: Johns Hopkins University Press, 1985); and Neil H. Wasserman, *From Invention to Innovation: Long-Distance Telephone Transmission at the Turn of the Century* (Baltimore: Johns Hopkins University Press, 1985).
5. For the central examples cited here, see Alan S. Russell, "Pitfalls and Pleasures in New Aluminum Process Development," *Metallurgical Transactions*, vol. 12B (June 1981). pp. 203–215; and Margaret B.W. Graham, *The Business of Research: RCA and the Videodisc* (New York: Cambridge University Press, in press). See also Bettye H. Pruitt and George D. Smith, "The Corporate Management of Innovation: Alcoa Research, Aircraft Alloys, and the Problem of Stress Corrosion Cracking," *Research on Technological Innovation, Management and Policy*, vol. 3 (New York: JAI Press, in press) for more extensive coverage of R&D management at Alcoa.
6. See William Abernathy, Kim Clark and Alan Kantrow, "The New Industrial Competition," *Harvard Business Review*, September–October 1981. Loss of technological edge is reflected in assessments by experts in many industries of the US position relative to the Japanese and in the declining interest of foreign licensees to pay for American technology. Such developments in the 1980s may be traceable to the de-emphasis on long-term R&D that occurred in the 1970s. According to Louis B. Fleming of *The Los Angeles Times* in his *Boston Globe* article (October 31, 1982) entitled "The US Backslide in R&D," R&D as a percentage of GNP declined from nearly 3% in the mid-1960s to just over 2% in the early 1980s, and all but 5% of industrial R&D money over the past decade has been focused on short-term, productivity-oriented work.
7. Richard S. Rosenbloom and Alan M. Kantrow, "The Nurturing of Corporate Research," *Harvard Business Review*, January–February 1982. See also Richard F. Hirsh, "Note on Research and Development in the United States" (1983), and "Note on Industrial Support of Basic Research" (1984), Harvard Business School.
8. Lowell W. Steele, *Innovation in Big Business* (New York: Elsevier, 1975).
9. See Edwin Mansfield, *The Economics of Technological Change* (New York: W.W. Norton, 1968). Chapter 3, "Industrial Research and Development," gives in-depth coverage of these statistics.
10. See Margaret B.W. Graham, "Industrial Research in the Age of Big Science," *op. cit.*
11. Richard Hirsh, "Note on Industrial Research and Development" (Harvard Business School, 1983) provides a useful summary of voluminous data from the National Science Foundation.
12. See Edwin Mansfield, *The Economics of Technological Change*, Chapter 3, *op. cit.*
13. In 1962, Ph.D.s in physics commanded salaries of $18,000 on the average, while the average Ph.D. in chemistry received $16,000. Even the latter figure was several thousand dollars above the average for other fields. See Graham, "Industrial Research in the Age of Big Science," *op. cit.*, p. 58.
14. Walter McDougall, *The Heavens and the Earth* (New York: Basic Books, 1985) maintains that the US humiliation over Sputnik was popularly interpreted as a failure of US science, even though engineering was

really the discipline most involved, and political considerations were decisive in determining which country actually lifted the first round hunk of metal into orbit.

15. See Nelson and Langlois, "Industrial Innovation Policy: Lessons from American History," *op. cit.*, p. 815.

16. See Alan S. Russell, "Pitfalls and Pleasures in New Aluminum Process Development," *op. cit.*

17. It should be noted that the prohibition against package licensing did not apply to overseas licensing, and in the late 1950s RCA adopted a very profitable practice of licensing its leading-edge electronics technology in Japan and Europe that was to last for nearly 30 years.

18. See Baker, Bean *et al.*, "R&D in Corporate Strategic Planning," *op. cit.*; Rolf Piekarz, "R&D and Productivity Growth: Policy Studies and Issues," AEA Papers and Proceedings, vol. 73, no. 2; Robert A. Burgelman, "Managing the Internal Corporate Venturing Process," *Sloan Management Review*, Vol. 5, no. 2 (Winter 1982).

19. See Robert A. Burgelman, "Designs for Corporate Entrepreneurship in Established Firms," *California Management Review* (1984) for two different views of the way strategy is actually formulated.

20. The Baker, Bean *et al.* study of innovation over 200 companies has confirmed this point, finding that the most significant innovations originating with R&D had a low degree of involvement with primary users and a high degree of involvement with general management, mostly outside the formal planning process. See Baker, Bean *et al.*, "R&D in Corporate Strategic Planning," *op. cit.*, p. 83.

21. Piekarz, "R&D Productivity Increases," AEA Papers and Proceedings, cites the National Science Foundation's program to set up joint university-industry centers in domains of applied science and the Stevenson-Wydler Act of 1980 to extend it. He also notes the Bayh-Dole Act of 1980 to permit certain research-performing groups to retain title to patents to federally funded research in pursuit of better commercialization.

22. See "R&D Funds from Federal Support," *Academic Science/Engineering: 1972–83* (Washington, DC: US Government Printing Office, 1984), p. 5.

23. See National Science Board, *University-Industry Research Relationships: Myths, Realities and Potentials*, 14th Annual Report of the National Science Board (Washington, DC: US Government Printing Office, 1983), p. 28.

24. For a comprehensive discussion of different approaches to innovation, see Edward B. Roberts, "New Ventures for Corporate Growth," *Harvard Business Review*, July–August 1980.

25. See John Friar and Mel Horwitch, "The Current Transformation of Technology Strategy: The Attempt to Create Multiple Avenues for Innovation within the Large Corporation," MIT Sloan School Working Paper 1618-84, December 20, 1984.

26. Wesley M. Cohen and David C. Mowery, "Firm Heterogeneity and R&D: An Agenda for Research" in Bozeman, Crow and Link, *Strategic Management of Industrial R&D, op. cit.*, p. 121.

27. See Robert A. Burgelman, "Managing the Corporate Venturing Process" and Edward Roberts, "New Ventures for Corporate Growth," *op. cit.*

28. See Norman Fast, "The DuPont Development Department from 1960 to 1976" (Harvard Business School Note, 1977), and Norman Fast, "The Future of Industrial New Venture Departments," *Industrial Marketing Management* (1979), pp. 264–273.

29. Lowell W. Steele, *Innovation in Big Business, op. cit.*, p. 226.

Corporate Strategies
for Managing Emerging Technologies

William F. Hamilton

ABSTRACT. The emergence of radically new industrial technology is a powerful competitive force with significant strategic implications. Entirely new industries may develop around an emerging technology as existing industries are transformed or destroyed in its wake. Schumpeter[1] aptly characterized such technological change as a force of "creative destruction," which leaves both winners and losers among industrial firms. What factors distinguish these firms and their strategies for dealing with technological change? This paper reports on a study of the strategic options available to firms facing radical technological change, and the strategic choices made by firms involved in the emerging biotechnology field. Of particular interest are the widespread use of external relationships and their roles in the technology strategies of established firms. The paper begins with brief definitions of established and emerging firms, followed by a review of insights into the strategic nature of technological change drawn from prior studies. The evolving positions of established and emerging firms in the biotechnology field are then described with some elaboration of the collaborative relationships which characterize its early development. A conceptual framework is proposed to differentiate the strategic choices made by established firms in response to advances in biotechnology, and this framework is used to examine the roles played by selected interorganizational relationships in corporate strategies. The paper argues that these external alliances are appropriate initial responses to the strategic management challenges presented by radical technological change, but that the nature and significance of these alliances and associated corporate strategies change as the technology advances toward commercialization.

The distinction between established and emerging firms is an important one in the context of technological change. An emerging firm is one created to exploit a new technology. Such entrepreneurial firms typically focus their efforts narrowly on selected technical innovations and market niches. They face substantial financial, organizational and market hurdles in attempting to commercialize their technology and establish viable competitive positions. The emerging firms considered in this paper have developed since the early 1970s with the specific objective of extending

Dr. Hamilton is Director of the Management and Technology Program and Landau Professor of Management and Technology in the Wharton School and the School of Engineering and Applied Science at the University of Pennsylvania. His teaching and research interests include the management of technology and innovation with particular emphasis on the strategic management challenges and choices presented by technological change.

and exploiting advances in biotechnology through new commercial products and processes. These firms have played a significant role in the early technical and commercial development of the field.

Established firms, in contrast, are those with positions in existing technologies and markets at the time a new technology appears. These firms face threats to their existing businesses, strategies and structures, in addition to the new opportunities presented by advancing technology. The established firms of interest in this paper were active in such traditional industry sectors as pharmaceuticals, chemicals, energy and food processing before the recent period of major scientific and technical advances in biotechnology.

Strategic Dimensions of Technological Change

The strategic nature and implications of technology have received increasing attention in recent years. One of the earliest and most extensively studied areas is the role of technological change in economic growth. Despite difficulties in measurement and differences among studies, economists generally agree that technological advance has been a significant contributor to America's productivity growth and economic prosperity.[2] More recently, international competitive pressures have stimulated wide-ranging examination of high technology industries in the US and their future prospects.[3] The growing recognition of the strategic importance of technology has also been reflected in the management literature by a stream of articles dealing with the technology-strategy relationship.[4] Several general conclusions from this literature are particularly relevant here.

The Strategic Impact of Technological Change

Technological change is a major competitive force with important strategic implications for individual companies and entire industries. This is especially true for revolutionary or radical changes in technology, which often introduce discontinuities in the evolution of products, processes and markets. Dramatic shifts in industry structure and competitive positions can result as the traditional advantages of established firms are eroded under revised rules of competition. New firms and established firms entering new businesses play important roles in this process, exploiting scientific and technical advances to overcome or circumvent entry barriers.[5]

Patterns of Technological Change

Technologies evolve through successive stages of development characterized by different technical and commercial requirements. In general, technical turbulence and commercial uncertainty in the emerging stage limit early advances in cost-performance. Transistor technology, for example, developed relatively slowly at first because of various technical problems and limited initial market interest. As knowledge increases and critical uncertainties are resolved, these limitations are overcome, leading in the growth stage to rapid cost-performance improvements and widespread commercialization. Technological maturity in the third stage leads to diminishing rates of technical and commercial advance, increasing vulnerability to substitution pressures from competing technologies in earlier stages of development. The nature and timing of evolution patterns vary considerably across technologies, and life cycles may span many decades from emergence to maturity.[6]

Strategic Responses to Technological Change

New technologies, particularly product technologies, are frequently introduced by firms outside traditional industry boundaries. Instant photography, for example, was commercialized by an emerging firm with no apparent connection to the conventional photographic industry. Synthetic fibers did not come from the textile industry, but from the chemical industry. In each case, the new technologies spawned products which offered improvements over existing products, created new business opportunities, and ultimately redefined traditional industry boundaries.

The strategic responses of established firms facing such technological changes may be offensive or defensive in nature. Offensive strategies are directed toward capitalizing on the opportunities offered by new technologies in order to enhance positions in existing businesses or diversify into new businesses. Defensive strategies are more focused on coping with the threats presented by technological change to established products and markets. Despite varied attempts to participate in the commercialization of new technologies in a variety of industries, few established firms seem to be able to manage this transition successfully.

The Emergence of Biotechnology[8]

Recent scientific and technical developments in recombinant DNA, tissue culture and supporting technologies present significant strategic management challenges and choices. Though only in its infancy, the biotechnology field gives every indication of great future potential. Dramatic technological advances in the past 12 years have generated intense international interest in the industrial application of living organisms. Continuing advances are expected to spawn significant new and improved products and processes in the pharmaceutical, agricultural, chemical and other industries. As a result, many observers anticipate that biotechnology will be a major source of economic growth in the next century. Rapid and widespread commercialization of biotechnology-derived products and processes are expected in the next few decades.

The strategic importance of this emerging technology is apparent. As noted in a recent study of international competitive positions in biotechnology, "companies or countries that lead in this developing field could gain a significant competitive edge over others because products are expected to be manufactured at lower cost, at higher purity, in larger quantities, and with decreased pollution and energy consumption."[9] The strategies by which key players position themselves in the technologies and markets associated with biotechnology's future will help to determine the ultimate winners in this international competition.

Broadly defined, biotechnology is "the application of biological organisms, systems or processes to manufacturing and service industries."[10] Biological organisms and processes have been applied throughout history in baking, brewing and agriculture. The appearance of antibiotics in the 1940s marked the increasing sophistication of the biological sciences, particularly microbiology, biochemistry, and microbial genetics. Since 1973, when the first gene was cloned successfully, attention has focused on the "new" generation of biotechnology, encompassing the techniques of genetic engineering, hybridomas and biochemical engineering (principally fermentation and large-scale cell culture). Dramatic scientific and technical advances have been made in these areas since 1973, and this rapid pace of technological change is expected to continue into the next century.[11]

Commercial Applications

The potential for commercial application of improved products and processes provides the driving force for continuing technical progress. In the long run, biotechnology could find applications in any industry involved with biological processes or in which biological processes might substitute for chemical processes. Pharmaceuticals, agriculture and industrial chemicals are the industrial sectors most often identified as primary targets of biotechnology applications in the next 15 years.

In pharmaceuticals and health care, biotechnology applications are expected to improve the quality and efficacy of existing products, expand production of known compounds not now available in commercially significant quantities, and create entirely new therapeutics, diagnostics and drug delivery systems. These developments may bring dramatic improvements in the diagnosis and treatment of cancer and cardiovascular and immunological diseases, among others. Although only a few biotechnology-derived products have reached the market, significant commercial payoffs are expected by the early 1990s.

Both animal and plant agriculture will benefit from new biotechnology-derived products and processes. In addition to improved animal vaccines, diagnostics, hormones and drugs, biotechnology will ultimately offer the capability to alter the genetic structures of cattle and other animals to improve quality and increase productivity. Similarly, genetically engineered seeds and bacteria will increase yields, improve quality, and expand potential cultivation regions for many important crops. Recent advances in agricultural applications have exceeded earlier expectations, and significant commercial activity should be achieved by the mid-1990s.

Industrial chemicals, particularly specialty chemicals and food additives, represent another major opportunity for biotechnology applications. Improvements in current bioprocessing methods (*e.g.*, amino acid production) and replacement of current chemical processes by new and far more efficient bioprocesses can result in lower costs and greater flexibility in the production of a vast array of organic chemicals. While potentially quite significant, the commercial impact of biotechnology on industrial chemicals will probably not be realized until the late 1990s.

These and many other potential commercial applications of biotechnology are indeed impressive. The wide-ranging possibilities and inherent uncertainties, however, have produced widely divergent market projections for new products and processes. Forecasts of the worldwide market for biotechnology-derived products, compiled by the US Department of Commerce, for example, range from $15 billion to more than $100 billion by the year 2000.[12] Estimates of the future impact of increased productivity in the industrial processes through biotechnology are considerably more difficult to make.

The direction and rate of continued progress in these and other commercial applications will depend on a number of factors, including the evolving nature of the biotechnology field itself. In considering this evolution, it is important to resist the temptation to characterize biotechnology as an "industry." At this early stage in its development, biotechnology represents a set of techniques with potential application and strategic impact in a number of established industries, some of which will no doubt undergo significant restructuring in the coming decades. Whether or not a new "biotechnology industry" will emerge remains to be seen.

Biotechnology Players

It has been estimated that the companies, institutes and universities involved in biotechnology number in the thousands worldwide. Several hundred US firms are actively involved in biotechnology research, development and commercialization through both internal programs and collaborative relationships with other organizations.

The most dynamic participants are the small, pioneering biotechnology firms, which have emerged since the early 1970s with the support of venture capital and corporate investors. Cetus and Genentech are generally considered among the leaders in this group.[13] These emerging firms combined scientific talents from leading academic research laboratories with a vision of commercial opportunities that excited the investment community in the early 1980s. When Genentech went public in 1980, its share price soared from an initial $35 to $89 in less than an hour. Cetus followed five months later with an initial public offering that raised $115 million, setting a Wall Street record. By the end of 1981, 30 emerging biotechnology firms had raised $500 million through a combination of public and private financing. Approximately 150 start-up biotechnology companies have emerged in the US, representing a total investment of between $3 and $4 billion.[14] This infusion of funds has vastly increased the level of biotechnology research and development activities. It has also greatly increased the pressures on many emerging firms to deliver commercial products and processes.

Established firms have moved more slowly into biotechnology, but their commitments are growing as potential applications become more apparent. For the most part, these are large, multiproduct companies with product capabilities and market positions in industrial sectors likely to be affected directly by biotechnology-derived products and processes. Baxter-Travenol, Hoffman-La Roche, Johnson & Johnson, Lilly, Schering-Plough and SmithKline are among the many pharmaceutical and health-care firms with biotechnology programs; American Cyanamid, W.R. Grace, Koppers and Martin Marietta have supported biotechnology research directed at agricultural applications; and two chemical industry giants, duPont and Monsanto, have made biotechnology commitments spanning the pharmaceutical, agricultural and chemical sectors.

For many of these firms, biotechnology offers the potential for new and improved products and processes in existing lines of business. This appears to be the primary focus for most pharmaceutical firms. Other established firms like duPont, Corning, Monsanto and Shell are looking to advances in biotechnology for diversification opportunities.

Not surprisingly, the nature and level of participation by established firms in biotechnology varies from company to company. Some large companies are making major internal commitments to biotechnology. Monsanto and duPont, for example, recently opened new corporate laboratories for biotechnology research and development. A number of pharmaceutical firms are also reported to be supporting significant internal biotechnology programs, but this appears to be less common in other sectors.

Far more common are various types of collaborative relationships, which established firms have developed with emerging biotechnology firms and research organizations as vehicles for their participation in the field. These relationships number in the hundreds. As illustrated in Table 1 and in the following discussion, both the

TABLE 1. Selected collaborative relationships in biotechnology

ESTABLISHED FIRM	OTHER ORGANIZATION	NATURE OF RELATIONSHIP
Monsanto	Washington University	Research grant of $23.5 million for microbiology research. Monsanto retains exclusive patent rights.
Corning Glass, Eastman Kodak and Union Carbide	Cornell University	Research grant in which each corporation will provide $2.5 million in support over 6 years to support new biological institute and basic research programs in molecular genetics, cellular biology and cell production.
DuPont	Harvard University	Research grant of $6 million to support basic research in molecular genetics.
Hoffmann-LaRoche	Genentech	Research contracts for development of human interferon; agreement provides for manufacturing by both partners and marketing by Hoffmann-LaRoche.
H.J. Heinz	BioTechnica	R&D contracts to use genetic engineering techniques in development of manufacturing processes; BioTechnica will receive royalties based on future product sales.
Schering AG (West Germany)	Genex	R&D contracts for development of rDNA products for heart disease therapy and rDNA-based process technology; also provision for licensing arrangements.

TABLE 1 (Continued)

ESTABLISHED FIRM	OTHER ORGANIZATION	NATURE OF RELATIONSHIP
Shell Oil	Collaborative Research	Development contract under which Shell (via a subsidiary) will support clinical trials of CR's Interlevkin-2; CR will retain manufacturing rights and will receive royalties on product sales.
Johnson & Johnson	Bio Logicals	Licensing agreement for therapeutic agents and other unspecified healthcare products; J&J also has a 7% equity share in Bio Logicals.
Daiichi Seiyaku Co. (Japan)	Genetic Systems	Licensing agreement to market Genetic Systems diagnostic kits in Japan.
Abbott Laboratories	Centocor	Licensing agreement to co-market Centocor's cancer diagnostic products.
Dow Chemical	Collaborative Research	Equity investment (5%) of $5 million plus warrants to purchase an additional 5% for $1 million.
Kellogg	Agrigenetics	Equity investment of $10 million.
Lubrizol	Genentech	Equity investments initiated in 1979 through Lubrizol's venture capital group; holding has been increased to 20% for a total cost of $15 million.
Corning Glass Works	Genentech	Joint venture company, Genencor, formed to develop enzymes for food processing and chemical industries.
W.R. Grace	Cetus	Joint venture formed to develop new agricultural products, including higher yield, disease-resistant crops.
Kirin Brewery (Japan)	Applied Molecular Genetics	Joint venture for worldwide production and marketing of rDNA-derived product; Kirin will invest $12 million, while AMGen will provide technology and additional financial support for the venture.

Source: "Biotechnology—Seeking the Right Corporate Combinations," *Chemical Week*, September 30, 1981; Emily A. Arakaki, "A Study of the U.S. Competitive Position in Biotechnology," U.S. Department of Commerce, July 1984; *Commercial Biotechnology: An International Analysis*, U.S. Congress, Office of Technology Assessment, January 1984; Dean Witter Reynolds, Inc.

frequency and the variety of these linkages are impressive. Five principal forms of collaborative relationships in the biotechnology field can be identified for discussion purposes.

Research Grants. Many established corporations and some emerging corporations have funded research programs in broadly defined areas of interest at major university research laboratories and private research institutes. These may involve some research participation by scientists from the supporting firms, and often provide for exclusive licensing or patient rights. One of the largest commitments for research support was made by Monsanto in 1982, when it announced a $23.5 million grant to the Washington University Medical School for microbiology research. Company scientists participate in the selection and monitoring of research projects, and Monsanto retains patent rights. In another major research grant, Corning Glass, Eastman Kodak and Union Carbide have committed $7.5 million in support of a new research institute at Cornell University and basic research programs in molecular genetics, cellular biology, and cell production.

R&D Contracts. A wide variety of contractual relationships are used to support targeted research in specific technology and/or application areas. The nature and desired outcomes of the research are generally well specified, as are patent rights, developmental responsibilities, and commercialization arrangements. The funding firms often obtain exclusive licenses on any resulting products or processes, while their partners may retain rights to patents and royalties in addition to contract fees. For example, Bio Technica is using genetic engineering techniques to develop improved production processes under a contract with H.J. Heinz, which provides for royalties based on future product sales. Similarly, Genentech and Hoffman-La Roche entered into a contract for the development of human interferons; Hoffman-La Roche will commercialize the resulting products and Genentech will receive royalties on future sales.

Licenses. The rights to produce and market specific biotechnology-derived products have been transferred to established firms through both exclusive and non-exclusive licensing arrangements with emerging firms in return for royalty payments. Patented processes may also be licensed. Such licensing arrangements may be tied to other contractual or equity relationships or may be entirely separate transactions. Johnson & Johnson has a licensing arrangement with Bio Logicals for health-care products in addition to a 7% equity share; Abbott Laboratories will market selected Centocor diagnostic products in the US and Europe through a non-exclusive license.

Equity Investments. Acquiring equity in an emerging firm through direct purchase or as a result of contract or licensing fees is another path taken by a number of established firms seeking participation in biotechnology. Dow Chemical Company, for example, purchased a 5% equity share in Collaborative Research for $5 million in 1981 with an option to purchase an additional 5% share for $1 million. National Distillers owns an 11% share in Cetus, and Fluor, Lubrizol and Monsanto are among the equity investors in Genentech. In many cases, such equity purchases complement research and licensing relationships; in other cases (*e.g.*, Lubrizol's 20% share of Genentech) they are limited to venture investments with no additional participation by the established firms.

Joint Ventures. The most interesting form of collaborative relationship is the joint venture, generally reflected in the formation of a separate, jointly owned company with clearly defined commercialization objectives. For example, Genencor was formed by Corning Glass and Genentech in 1982 to develop industrial enzymes for chemical and food processing. Cetus and W.R. Grace initiated a 49%–51% joint venture in 1984 to develop selected new agricultural products.

Many established firms have collaborated with multiple partners in different application areas through a variety of relationships to broaden their chances of future technical and commercial success. While the overall level of biotechnology-related activity has increased in the past five years, interest in equity investments appears to have declined in favor of internal programs.

Strategic Options and Choices

The rapid emergence of biotechnology and the prospect of commercial applications present important strategic management challenges to established firms. Most face both opportunities and threats. Those with positions in businesses likely to feel the early impact of biotechnology applications may face direct challenges from substitute products and processes. In addition, new technology-driven business opportunities may have important strategic implications for firms in both related and unrelated businesses. Although the ultimate directions and payoffs are highly uncertain at this early stage, many established firms have chosen to participate in biotechnology development. Analysis of their strategies for managing this potentially important emerging technology can provide useful insights for other firms facing radical technological change.

Strategic Options

During the early evolution of a new technology, corporations may consider several different strategies for participation in its commercial development: [15]

Opening Windows. The initial objective of many established firms is to identify and monitor leading-edge technologies. This can greatly expand the knowledge base on which judgments are made about future technical developments, market opportunities, and commercialization requirements. Such an approach may involve internal programs (*e.g.*, exploratory research, technology monitoring, etc.) or external linkages (*e.g.*, research grants, equity investments) or both with primary emphasis on increased awareness and understanding of the emerging technology and its implications. This typically involves a limited commitment of resources, and permits broad scope and flexibility in technology and market coverage. A "window strategy" is most often useful in the very early stages of scientific and technical development.

Creating Options. The primary thrust of an "options strategy" is creation of defined opportunities for future active participation in emerging technologies and commercial applications. These may include internal development projects or external linkages (*e.g.*, contract research) or both with a focus on particular technical or market areas which offer the potential for increased involvement and resource commitment. This strategy implies greater investments of time and funds in fewer targeted developmental areas than does the window strategy.

Establishing Positions. Firms pursuing a "positioning strategy" are staking out their competitive positions in selected technologies and markets with the intention of continued commitments in these or related commercial arenas. In effect, they are exercising available options for active participation in the emerging technology. This strategy reflects even greater levels of commitment and focus than those discussed above.

The general progression of these technology strategies over time is illustrated in Figure 1. Applying this conceptual framework to the biotechnology field highlights

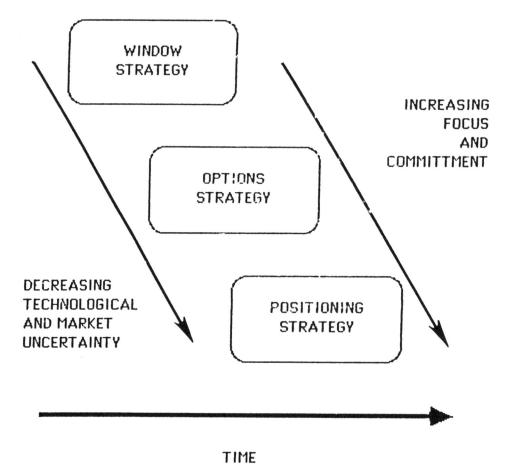

TIME

FIGURE 1. Progression of Technology Strategies

several apparent trends. First, there is a logical progression in strategic emphasis from information-gathering to more focused commitments as technologies and markets develop. The initial involvements of many established firms in the 1970s were clearly of an exploratory nature; as possibilities and requirements became more certain, some firms targeted particular technical advances and commercial applications for development; and, as these near commercialization status, greater commitments to fewer areas follow. When strong market positions or advanced technical developments exist, as in the Lilly-Genentech alliance to commercialize Humulin, firms may move directly to positioning commitments.

Some established firms are pursuing different technology strategies in different application areas. Where commercialization opportunities are more immediate, as is the case in pharmaceuticals, option or positioning strategies may be appropriate; in other areas, as in specialty chemicals production, a window strategy may be best. Monsanto's extensive portfolio of biotechnology programs reflects involvement in each stage of this technology strategy progression.

The Strategic Use of Alliances

As described above, the early evolution of the biotechnology field has been marked by extensive interorganizational relationships. Our research indicates that many of these cooperative arrangements play important roles in the technology strategies of the participating firms. Although this discussion is focused on established firms and their use of strategic alliances, a parallel analysis of the strategies and alliances pursued by emerging firms indicates that external alliances may play even more important roles in the strategies of these emerging firms.[16]

For the purposes of this study, a strategic alliance is defined as a formal linkage between firms which offers actual or potential strategic advantages to either or both firms. Such cooperative arrangements may take many forms, but all are based on two principal features: complementary strengths and mutual benefits.

In the biotechnology field, the vast majority of alliances have linked small, technology-driven, emerging companies and large, well-established companies with extensive manufacturing and marketing capabilities. For most emerging firms, these alliances provide the financial support necessary for continued scientific research, as well as access to important product development and marketing resources. Established firms, on the other hand, gain insights and access to the technical knowledge and skills of their partners. The benefits of successful alliances include expansion of the knowledge base available to both partners, a sharing of risks, and enhanced strategic positions in selected technologies and markets.[17]

The general pattern of alliances and associated strategies observed for established firms in the biotechnology field is summarized in Table 2. Research grants, minority equity investments, and exploratory research contracts are most supportive of the information-gathering objectives which characterize the window strategy. As interests become more defined, some combination of equity investments, targeted R&D contracts, licensing arrangements, and joint ventures may be used to develop and evaluate options in selected technical and commercial areas for possible major future commitments. Specific development contracts, often in conjunction with

TABLE 2. Principal strategic roles of alliances used by established firms

ALLIANCE	STRATEGY			COMMENTS
	WINDOW	OPTIONS	POSITIONING	
RESEARCH GRANT	✓			• Access to pioneering research • Limited proprietary benefits • Not appropriate for targeted R&D
R&D CONTRACT	✓	✓	✓	• Complement to internal R&D; minimal resource commitments • Limited control; transfer of technology difficult • Very flexible: focus can range from exploratory to commercialization; often linked to licensing arrangements
LICENSE		✓	✓	• Early access to new products/processes; limited initial investment • Dependence on others; long term costs may be high • Focus shifts from technical to market development
EQUITY	✓	✓		• Limited initial commitment required; some opportunity to influence R&D directions • Limited control; access to technology difficult • Often associated with R&D contracts/licensing arrangements; may lead to acquisition in long term
JOINT VENTURE		✓	✓	• Shared technical and commercial risks; takes full advantage of complementary strengths • Potential for conflict between partners; can require significant financial and personnel commitments • Focus shifts from development to commercialization

licensing arrangements, and joint ventures are most appropriate for positioning commitments.

Thus, the attractiveness of selected external alliances varies over time as technology strategies evolve. In addition, the nature and conditions of these alliances may also change somewhat with the changing strategies. Biotechnology R&D contracts, for example, may be loosely defined in early exploratory efforts, but more highly focused on specific product or process developments in later stages.

Another pattern observed in the biotechnology field is the increasing internal orientation reflected in the evolution of technology strategies. As uncertainties diminish and commercial opportunities become clearer over time, there are strong economic and managerial incentives to increase control over development programs and to reduce reliance on outside organizations. Moreover, the increased focus and commitment implied by options and positioning strategies typically demand higher levels of in-house expertise to ensure that the most appropriate technologies and markets are being pursued. The result is an apparent increase in the relative importance of internal — rather than external — programs.

Strategic Choices in Biotechnology

In summary, analysis of the emerging biotechnology field and the strategic choices made by a sample of established and emerging firms indicates that:

- Significant strategic challenges face both established and emerging firms seeking to participate in biotechnology. Rapid technological advances with wide-ranging, but still highly uncertain, commercial implications favor initial strategic choices, which limit risks and preserve future options.
- Several distinct strategies for managing this emerging technology are evident in the internal and external commitments made by established firms. These tend to evolve toward greater levels of commitment in more narrowly focused areas as technical and market uncertainties decline.
- Strategic alliances between established and emerging firms are widespread in biotechnology. However, the nature and strategic roles of these alliances are changing as the underlying technology and competitive environments change. Strategic alliances are particularly important in the earliest stages of technology development. Increasing strategic focus and commitment are likely to be reflected in greater relative emphasis on internal biotechnology programs.

The observations reported here are the preliminary findings of a continuing research program focused on the strategic challenges and choices presented by technological change. As biotechnology moves toward commercialization, the evolving strategies and shifting competitive positions of current and future participants are expected to reflect several trends:

- a continuing shift to internal programs and greater direct control of biotechnology activities by established firms with fewer external alliances of strategic importance;

- accelerating commitments of technical and financial resources as current developmental programs reach commercialization; and
- a decline in the number of emerging firms active in key biotechnology application areas as the requirements of commercialization and intense competitive pressures combine to favor established firms.

These are among the expectations which form the basis for continued monitoring and analysis of the emerging biotechnology field and the strategic behavior of participating firms.

General Implications for Corporate Strategy

A primary objective of the research reported in this paper is to learn more about how corporations capitalize on the strategic opportunities and/or cope with the strategic threats presented by technological change. This is a particularly important issue in industrial sectors likely to be affected by advances in artificial intelligence, VLSI, engineered materials and other emerging technologies. At least several general lessons for corporate strategy can be drawn from experiences to date in the biotechnology field:

- No single firm commands the full range of resources necessary to manage an emerging technology in its initial stages of development. Even the most successful established firms must therefore look to external sources if they wish to participate in commercializing the new technology.
- The strategies pursued by established firms in an emerging technology area will shift as the technology and associated markets develop, reflecting increased commitments to more focused programs over time. Firms planning to participate in an emerging technology should anticipate and organize to manage a rapid shift in strategic emphasis from opening windows to creating options and establishing positions.
- The strategic positions of established and emerging firms are highly complementary during the early development of a new technology, but the nature and significance of this "strategic complementarity" changes with shifting technology strategies. As a result, external alliances deserve careful consideration as mechanisms for managing radical technological change, but care must be taken to tailor these relationships to meet changing strategic requirements.

Of course, the strategic challenges and choices presented by emerging technologies differ from firm to firm and from industry to industry. Emerging technologies also differ in their nature, rates of development, commercial impact, and other important characteristics. The particular strategic choices made by firms in the biotechnology field may, therefore, be inappropriate for other firms in other contexts. Indeed, only the passage of time will reveal just how appropriate these choices have been in biotechnology.

Acknowledgments

I would like to thank Nancy Olson and Bernadette Fendrock for their assistance in the research reported in this article. I would also like to thank Richard Klavans and Graham Mitchell for their very helpful comments.

Notes

1. J.A. Schumpeter, *The Theory of Economic Development* (Cambridge, MA: Harvard University Press, 1934).
2. For example, see Edwin Mansfield, "Contribution of R&D to Economic Growth in the United States," *Science*, February 4, 1972; E.F. Denison, *Accounting for United States Economic Growth 1929–1969* (Washington, DC: The Brookings Institution, 1974); Simon Kuznets, "Technological Innovations and Economic Growth" in Patrick Kelly and Melvin Krantzberg, eds., *Technological Innovation: A Critical Review of Current Knowlege* (San Francisco: San Francisco Press, 1978); and J.W. Kendrick, *Sources of Growth in Real Product and Productivity in Eight Countries, 1960–1978* (New York: Office of Economic Research, New York Stock Exchange, 1981).
3. Robotics, computers, semiconductors and telecommunications were the initial subjects of a series on "High Technology Industries: Profiles and Outlooks" by the International Trade Administration, US Department of Commerce, April 1983; a subsequent study on the competitive outlook for biotechnology appeared in the same series in July 1984.
4. For example, see Alan M. Kantrow, "The Strategy-Technology Connection," *Harvard Business Review*. July–August 1980; Michael E. Porter, "The Technological Dimension of Competitive Strategy" in Richard S. Rosenbloom, ed., *Research on Technological Innovation, Management and Policy* (Greenwich, CT: JAI Press, 1983); and Alan L. Frohman, "Putting Technology Into Strategy," *Journal of Business Strategy*, Spring 1985.
5. Edwin Mansfield *et al.*, *The Production and Application of New Industrial Technology* (New York: W.W. Norton, 1977), p. 16; and Michael E. Porter, "Technology and Competitive Advantage," *Journal of Business Strategy*, Winter 1985.
6. For a discussion and examples of the technology life-cycle, see Philip A. Roussel, "Technological Maturity Proves a Valid and Important Concept," *Research Management*, January–February 1984; more complex models of technological evolution are suggested in James M. Utterback and William J. Abernathy, "A Dynamic Model of Product and Process Innovation," *Omega*, Vol. 9, no. 4; C. de Bresson and J. Townsend, "Multi-Variate Models for Innovation—Looking at the Abernathy-Utterback Model with Other Data," *Omega*, Vol. 9, no. 4 (1981); and Devendra Sahal, *Patterns of Technological Innovation* (Reading, MA: Addison-Wesley, 1981).
7. See, for example, Arnold C. Cooper and Dan Schendel, "Strategic Responses to Technological Threats," *Business Horizons*, February 1976, for a study of seven industries challenged by new technologies; see also Chapter VI, "Technological Change in U.S. Industry" in Donald A. Schon, *Technology and Change* (New York: Delacorte Press, 1967) for his analysis of "innovation by invasion" in the textile, machine tool, and building industries.
8. Biotechnology was chosen as the context for research into corporate strategies for managing emerging technologies because of the revolutionary nature of the technological changes in progress, the wide range of industries likely to be affected, and the rich variety of strategies being pursued by present and potential participants. Two broad questions guide the research:

    1. What strategic options are available to firms facing technological change?
    2. What factors influence the responses of established and emerging firms to new technologies?

    The current phase of the study draws on three primary data sources: an industry database on firms participating in biotechnology and their commitments to selected technologies and markets; in-depth case studies of a sample of five established and five emerging firms with biotechnology involvement; and interviews with managers in the sample firms. In total, these ten firms are involved in more than 80 formal collaborative relationships with other firms and research organizations.
9. Emily A. Arakaki, "A Study of the U.S. Competitive Position in Biotechnology" in *High-Technology Industries: Profiles and Outlooks—Biotechnology* (Washington, DC: International Trade Administration, US Department of Commerce, July 1984), p. 52.
10. This is one of a number of definitions reported in *Biotechnology: International Trends and Perspectives* (Paris: Organization for Economic Cooperation and Development, 1982).

11. For extensive reviews of past developments and future prospects in the biotechnology field, see *Commercial Biotechnology: An International Analysis* (Washington, DC: Office of Technology Assessment, US Congress, January 1984); and Emily A. Arakaki, "A Study of the U.S. Competitive Position in Biotechnology," *op. cit.*

12. Emily A. Arakaki, "A Study of the U.S. Competitive Position in Biotechnology," *op. cit.*

13. For a current assessment of the leadership positions and strategies of Cetus and Genentech, see "Corporate Strategies—and Then There Were Two," *Biotechnology*, July 1985.

14. Ralph W.F. Hardy and David J. Glass, "Our Investment: What Is at Stake?" *Issues in Science and Technology*, Spring 1985.

15. Attention in this paper is focused on firms with some involvement—if not major commitments—in an emerging technology. No consideration will be given here to the extremely important issues surrounding the decision to participate.

16. William F. Hamilton, Nancy Olson and Bernadette Fendrock, "Strategic Challenges and Choices in Biotechnology," Management and Technology Program, University of Pennsylvania, June 1985.

17. For an overview of interfirm relationships and analysis of joint venture activities and strategies in a number of industrial sectors, see Sanford V. Berg, Jerome Duncan and Philip Friedman, *Joint Venture Strategies and Corporate Innovation* (Cambridge, MA: Oelgeschlager, Gunn & Hain, 1982); also see John Friar and Mel Horwitch, "The Current Transformation of Technology Strategy: The Attempt to Create Multiple Avenues for Innovation Within the Large Corporation," MIT Sloan School of Management, December 1984; and Edward B. Roberts and Charles A. Berry, "Entering New Businesses: Selecting Strategies for Success," *Sloan Management Review*, Spring 1985, for discussions of various cooperative relationships and their implications for corporate strategy.

Strategy and Technology
in the Toppan Printing Company

Kiyoshi Kinami

ABSTRACT. Although a mature industry, the printing industry has always been and is now in reality a technology-intensive sector. Technology strategy is now a key element in a large printing company's success. Toppan Printing Company is one such large firm. It is based in Japan, and it has continually grown during the postwar period. Toppan's strategy combines close attention to customer needs, upstream and downstream integration, and diversification into related business areas. A major ingredient in Toppan's success is an intense and high-level commitment to technology. Technological innovation is an essential part of practically all parts of its business. Of particular importance is the growing role of electronics and computer-based systems in Toppan's products and processes. Toppan is participating in and is anticipating strategically a post-industrial, information-based age.

Printing is often seen as a mature industry. It is certainly an old industry. The invention of movable-type printing by Gutenberg was undoubtedly one of the most significant inventions of the Renaissance period, along with gunpowder and the compass. As Victor Hugo observed, the invention of printing by movable type destroyed the authority of the cathedral, a symbol of the medieval age, and acted as a bridge to the modern age. The knowledge of letters and the use of letters that was once the property of a privileged few (kings and priests) became the property of the populace. In fact, printing can also be viewed as a modern technology-intensive industry where innovation is a key factor in continued success.

Printing is really the mass medium for reproducing and communicating information in the form of characters and images. As such, the industry has become extremely diversified. Printing is used for interior decoration materials, such as wood-grain printing, clothing, and packages. Moreover, advanced printing techniques are now applied in the production of precision electronic components, such as photomasks of patterns for integrated electronic circuits, multi-layer printed circuit boards, and color filters built into video cameras. Increasing attention is now being given to new forms of information systems, called "new media," such as ISDN (integrated circuit digitalized network) that uses fiber-optics, CATV (cable television service), and Videotex. These new breakthroughs in developing techniques for

Kiyoshi Kinami is Senior Managing Director of the Toppan Printing Company. He has overall responsibility for production, R&D, and engineering. Mr. Kinami has worked for Toppan since 1946, and has held a wide variety of positions within the firm. He is a graduate of the Tokyo Institute of Technology.

achieving the successful merger of printing technology with information processing and telecommunications, are aimed at the complete utilization of information through the systematization of the storage processing and transmission of character and graphic data. These developments will certainly revolutionize the concept of printing itself.

This article discusses how one firm, Toppan Printing Company, explicitly uses technology throughout its corporate strategy in an attempt to stay at the forefront of this truly fast-changing industry.

An Overview of Toppan

There are approximately 36,000 firms engaged in the printing and related industries in Japan, of which approximately 3% have more than 200 employees. Most of these firms confine their activities to particular niches, and only a few firms, including Toppan, have the ability to provide a comprehensive range of printing and related services. Toppan estimates that it accounts for approximately 10% of total gross sales of the Japanese printing industry.

Toppan competes with its major rivals in practically all facets of the printing business, and also with many small printers whose particular strength has been in small-job lots. Toppan tries to provide for all the printing needs of its customers. In addition, Toppan believes that its emphasis on the development of new and specialized printing and related technology, on planning and research to find new applications of printing technology, and on extensive investment in machinery and equipment have significantly contributed to its success. This experience has led Toppan to conclude that firms with greater financial, human and technological resources will continue to have competitive advantages over smaller firms. For example, the introduction by Toppan of a computerized type-setting system for Japanese characters, which automates the printing process and reduces printing costs, has enabled Toppan to compete effectively with small printing firms.

Toppan has an extensive product line. The company competes with its major competitors and other specialized manufacturers for sales of precision electronic components. The firm is one of the two major suppliers in Japan of video-camera color filters and photomasks (although there are numerous suppliers in Japan of printed circuitry), IC lead frames, and parts of fluorescent indicator tubes. Toppan provides a full range of design and manufacturing services for packaging materials other than glass and metal. Such services are provided by only one other firm in Japan, although there are numerous specialized suppliers of packaging materials produced by Toppan and its subsidiaries. Finally, interior decor materials are also produced by Toppan.

Toppan was founded, with its head office in Tokyo, in January 1900, and has been incorporated as a joint stock company under the laws of Japan since 1908. From the beginning, technology was a key element of Toppan's strategy. The firm began its business operations with what was then the very latest in printing technology, such as the letterpress, galvanograph, and intaglio printing techniques, which until then had not been utilized in Japan by other than the Printing Bureau of the Ministry of Finance. Toppan's first operations included the printing of cigarette packets. Its business soon expanded to the printing of other packages, books, maps, and other commercial jobs. Above all, Toppan's advanced technology enabled it to become the leading printer in the private sector of securities, bank notes, and paper currency. Business growth continued until World War II, during which virtually all commercial printing in Japan ceased, and a significant number of Toppan's printing facilities were destroyed.

Soon after the war, Toppan resumed operations in its remaining facilities, and secured an order for the printing of new yen bills from the government. With its long experience and expertise in printing, Toppan was well placed to take advantage of the recovery in the Japanese economy, and sales have continued to increase. Toppan is one of the two largest printing companies in Japan and one of the largest in the world.

Toppan has a consistent record of financial success. Fiscal 1984 represented Toppan's 32nd consecutive year of solid financial achievement, maintaining its position among Japan's top 100 companies. As seen in Figure 1, Toppan is capitalized at $98.7 million, and its net sales in fiscal 1984 reached $2.3 billion, an 8.9% increase over the previous year. Net income rose 7%, reaching $69 million. The company has 9,500 employees on its payroll in its 51 offices and 15 plants in Japan.

Toppan has continued to emphasize the importance of technology in its strategy. The company gradually diversified its business into other related areas, utilizing its printing, etching and photoengraving technologies. In 1952, using technology obtained under license, Toppan began printing on cellophane, aluminum, plastic and other materials. Applying this technology, the firm began manufacturing interior decor materials in 1958, and its business today also includes printing on cloth. The company also manufactures various packaging materials. In 1960, Toppan started production of precision electronic components. Today it is among the leading manufacturers in Japan of photomasks for ICs, including LSIs and VLSIs, IC lead frames, multi-layer printed circuit boards, video-camera color filters, and parts of fluorescent indicator tubes. In 1984, Toppan started to manufacture high-resolution shadowmasks for CRT terminals.

During the past 10 fiscal years, Toppan has constructed three new plants, has acquired one company in Japan, and has made further investments in its existing plants.

Toppan has also moved overseas. It opened representative offices in London in 1971 and in Duesseldorf in 1983. Overseas manufacturing subsidiaries or affiliates were established in Hong Kong in 1963, in Singapore in 1968, in the United States in 1971, and in Indonesia in 1973. Sales subsidiaries were established in Australia in 1974 and in the United Kingdom in 1983.

The Business Activities of Toppan

In order to understand Toppan's overall strategy — and especially the key role technology plays in it — let us first review briefly each of the firm's major business activities, as seen in Figure 2.

FINANCIAL HIGHLIGHTS
(Years ended May 31, 1984 and 1983)

	1984	1983
		(¥232=U.S.$1 as of May 31, 1984)
Paid-up capital	98,793,000	97,552,000
Net sales	2,289,108,000	2,101,810,000
Net income	69,224,000	64,707,000
Share in paid-up capital	70.07%	66.33%
Share in net sales	3.02%	3.08%
Cash dividends declared	16,811,000	15,961,000
Total assets	1,463,138,000	1,312,306,000
Long-term indebtedness	51,707,000	25,073,000
Shareholders' equity	715,767,000	650,694,000
Number of common stocks	458,370,624	452,639,777
Number of shareholders	38,809	38,970
Number of employees	9,453	8,983

Paid-up capital   In thousands of U.S. dollars

Year	Value
1980	78,427
1981	82,397
1982	88,681
1983	97,552
1984	98,793

(scale: 0, 10,000, 20,000, 30,000, 40,000, 50,000, 60,000, 70,000, 80,000, 90,000, 100,000)

Net sales   In millions of U.S. dollars

Year	Value
1980	1,567
1981	1,777
1982	1,929
1983	2,102
1984	2,289

(scale: 0, 200, 400, 600, 800, 1,000, 1,200, 1,400, 1,600, 1,800, 2,000, 2,200, 2,400)

Net income   In millions of U.S. dollars

Year	Value
1980	57
1981	59
1982	62
1983	65
1984	69

(scale: 0, 5, 10, 15, 20, 25, 30, 35, 40, 45, 50, 55, 60, 65, 70)

Net income per 100 shares   In U.S. dollars

Year	Value
1980	14.50
1981	13.95
1982	14.46
1983	14.29
1984	15.19

(scale: 0, 2.00, 4.00, 6.00, 8.00, 10.00, 12.00, 14.00, 16.00)

FIGURE 1. Toppan Printing Company.

Source: Annual Report, 1984

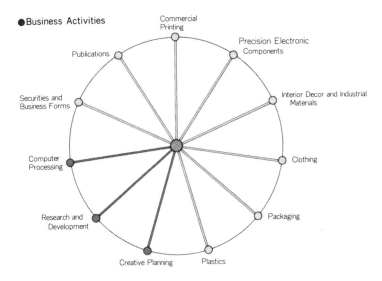

FIGURE 2. The business activities of Toppan.

Securities Printing

This category, which is one of Toppan's oldest lines of business, includes the printing of share and bond certificates, checks, bank deposit certificates and passbooks, bond and other credit cards, and lottery tickets. Toppan's long experience in securities printing has enabled it to obtain a leading position in the Japanese securities printing market. It is one of the few companies in Japan with the facilities for printing share certificates and bonds that meet the prescribed standards of the Tokyo Stock Exchange and other stock exchanges. Technology has also influenced this business segment. Toppan, in a joint venture with TDK Corporation, applies magnetic printing technology to the production of bank passbooks and credit cards, and is one of the two major suppliers of such products in Japan. In addition, in 1983, Toppan developed an "intelligent" card, incorporating an integrated circuit, which can carry several hundred times more information than magnetic strip cards. As the cashless economy approaches, plastic cards of all kinds will play an increasingly key role in daily life and in Toppan's operations.

Commercial Printing

Toppan produces a wide range of products in this category, such as posters, catalogs, leaflets, calendars, and commercial displays. In some cases, these products are marketed with the assistance of Toppan's planning and customer-aid activities. Customers include leading manufacturers of consumer goods in various fields and retailers. Also included in this category is the sale of printing-related equipment, including computerized control devices, platemaking machines, and plotters. Commercial printing accounted for approximately 25% of Toppan's nonconsolidated net sales for the fiscal year ending May 31, 1983.

Books and Magazines

Toppan prints a variety of books, including textbooks, dictionaries, reference books, art books, magazines, journals, paperback books, telephone directories, and other publications. Although Toppan's printing operations include platemaking, printing, binding and delivery to distributors and publishers, in common with most other large Japanese printers, Toppan does not engage in publishing. Again, technology is important for this business activity. In order to meet the constant demand for quicker printing with higher quality, Toppan has developed printing methods that utilize electronics and computer technology to achieve better performance. Such technological developments include a computerized type-setting system for Japanese characters, which is also used for other areas of printing.

Packaging Materials

Toppan is one of the leading producers of packaging material in Japan. The firm produces a wide range of packaging materials from paper and flexible packaging to plastic containers for various uses. Toppan also sells packaging machines. Customers include manufacturers of processed food, confectioneries, beverages, toiletries, cosmetics, pharmaceuticals, and medical supplies, and Toppan works in close cooperation with them. For example, where it is necessary to preserve the quality of packaged contents and to protect them from contamination, such as in the food, pharmaceutical and medical supply fields, Toppan manufactures packaging materials in hygienically controlled, germ-free production facilities.

Precision Electronic Components

Using a strategy that may distinguish it from large printing companies in other parts of the world, Toppan consciously applied its printing, etching and photoengraving technologies with the aim of entering the electronics field. The company now produces various components, including photomasks for the production of ICs, such as LSIs and VLSIs (16 kilobits and 64 kilobits), multi-layer printed circuit boards, IC lead frames, video-camera color filters, parts of fluorescent indicator tubes, and high-resolution shadow masks for CRT terminals. For the production of precision electronic components, Toppan utilizes advanced technologies, such as laser-beam engraving, computer-aided design and pattern generation, and high-speed, quality mass-production systems. In the production of semiconductors, the firm cooperates closely with semiconductor manufacturers in the design of circuitry. Production is carried out in special facilities where there is strict control of environment, temperature, humidity and vibration. Precision electronic components accounted for approximately 10% of Toppan's nonconsolidated net sales for the fiscal year ending May 31, 1983.

Interior Decor Materials and Other Miscellaneous Products

Toppan's etching and photoengraving technology has enabled the firm to reproduce patterns from natural materials for use on interior panels, floor surfaces, wallpaper and ceilings. The company manufactures several types of interior decor and building materials, placing emphasis on the development of heat-durable and lightweight materials. Extensive use is made of research that is carried out at the Toppan Interior Design Center, established in 1974. Interior decor materials accounted for approximately 10% of Toppan's nonconsolidated net sales for the fiscal year ending May 31, 1983.

Toppan's Current Strategy

Toppan, therefore, has actively accepted the challenge of participating in the sophisticated information age that is just starting to dawn. It is confident of its growing accumulation of relevant expertise. Responding to this changing competitive environment, Toppan's current strategy emphasizes the following elements.

Upstream Strategy, Downstream Strategy

The Japanese printing industry began to undertake an upstream strategy beginning in the late 1950s, and this upstream thrust now includes packaging, building materials, and the design of photomasks for ICs and LSIs. Moreover, this upstream strategy has naturally been accompanied by downstream strategy, which encompasses, for example, the insertion, wrapping, distribution and delivery of a package. Great attention is placed on fulfilling customer orders and meeting customer needs. The printing company must, first of all, ensure on-schedule delivery of orders. In addition, however, Toppan continually upgrades production control technology and, by doing so, more precisely meets the demands of its clients. Indeed, Toppan very actively works together with its clients, taking part in the initial planning and cooperating in their marketing activities. In this fashion, Toppan at times has been instrumental in opening up new markets for its customers.

The Toppan Idea Center

The "Toppan Idea Center" (TIC) was established in 1961 to promote Toppan's business through assistance to customers in the marketing planning of their products. TIC plans marketing strategy, undertakes market research, and assists in the development of new products, as well as producing sales promotion aids, such as video films, graphic designs, photographic camera works, give-aways, and novelties. TIC designs packaging materials, retail displays, and other items. TIC also plans and designs exhibitions, shows, and featured events. Toppan often participates in all phases of its customers' marketing planning — from the initial stages of production through to the commencement of actual sales. For these services, Toppan sometimes receives remuneration in the form of added value to the products or services. Toppan believes that the activities of TIC are important for developing close relationships between Toppan and its customers.

New technology can play a key role in such planning and customer-aid activities. In carrying out consumer buying trend surveys, for example, the Toppan Group Response Analysis systems uses computers which instantly tabulate survey data or display data in graphics. Or, to take another example, Toppan's packaging division utilizes a computerized package design system, which can tailor this task to manufacturers' specific needs.

The Total Media Development Institute Co., Ltd.

As part of its effort to help plan and design the theme pavilion of the Japanese government for an international exposition that was held in Osaka in 1970, Toppan established the Total Media Development Institute Co., Ltd., in September 1970. Since then, the Institute's scope has expanded. It took charge of the government theme pavilions at the Okinawa Ocean Expo and Tsukuba Expo '85. It plans, it designs, and it creates various kinds of media and design imagery for cultural institutions like the National Ethnology Museum and the National History Museum. Toppan believes that this activity provides Toppan with a highly refined and accumulated information base. The advanced and interdisciplinary engineering ability of the Total Media Institute functions as a key strategic think-tank that is one of the big mainstays that will help Toppan to survive as a true knowledge-based enterprise.

The CTS System

The Japanese language — unlike the 26-letter English alphabet — is composed of ten thousand kanji, or characters, which traditionally made type-setting for various lists, directories, dictionaries and indices troublesome, time-consuming and tedious. The introduction of computer-based technology, however, has significantly changed this situation. For 20 years, Toppan has been devoted to developing and utilizing this innovation. It has developed its Computerized Typesetting System (CTS), making possible computerized manuscript preparation, arrangement, automatic composition of indices, and proof-reading, as depicted in Figure 3. Toppan regards CTS as a key ingredient in the diversification of its printing-related technology.

The implications of CTS are enormous, and even now they are by no means fully realized. CTS can process large quantities of data, which enhances its ability to meet a wide variety of needs in business and industrial applications. Toppan has developed a universal character code conversion process, so that CTS can receive input from practically all types of word processors and terminals. Toppan is now able to provide publishing companies instantly with a variety of information, or to print by directly connecting Toppan with the computers of publishing companies. Indeed, CTS is also becoming an important data base.

The firm also owns the Toppan Scan-Note System, which is a computerized music-score output system.

CTS is closely connected to Toppan's Layout and Editing System, as depicted in Figure 4. Image information, such as photographs, characters, logos, etc., are read by an image scanner and similar equipment, and then registered in a computer. The designer can retrieve such images on the graphic display and create layouts and designs using the full range of functions of the display, including enlargement, reduction, revolution, shifting, and reproduction. This activity can be a large-volume, high-speed, and multi-operation system task, occasionally taking the form

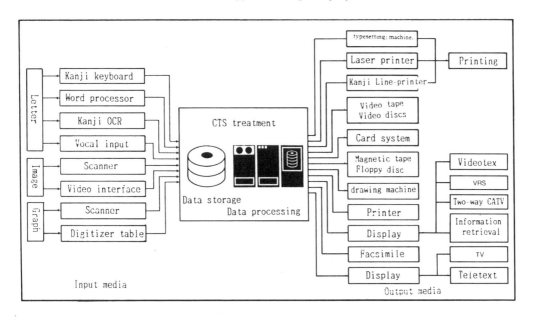

FIGURE 3. Flow of Toppan CTS system.

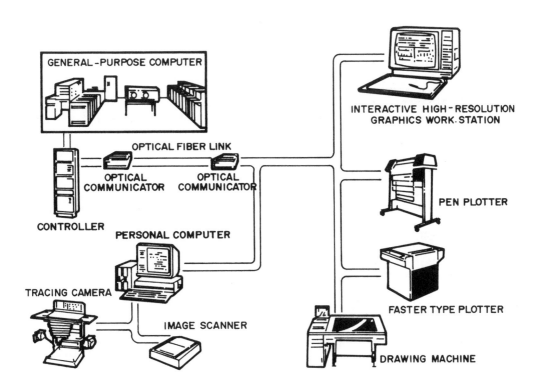

FIGURE 4. Layout and editing system.

of a LAN (Local Area Network) with terminals installed in Toppan design rooms or in clients' rooms. Platemaking can then take place automatically, using computerized pen-plotters and drawing and cutting machines.

Toppan's advanced character and graphic data processing technology is being combined with the introduction of all forms of telecommunications technology. This will help not only the company and its customers, but will result in linking affiliated companies, sales offices, production plants, suppliers, and others. It will also lead to the formation of a comprehensive digital network most suited to the advanced information society.

Precision Electronics

Toppan's most obvious high-technology activities are in the area of precision electronics, including integrated circuits, large-scale integrated circuits, and very large-scale integrated circuits. At first glance, one is apt to wonder why a printing company manufactures precision electronic components. But, since its invention in the 15th century, printing has been associated with high precision. Today's color print images are made up of a complicated overlapping of yellow, magenta, cyan and black colors in minute dots, ranging from a few microns to 100 microns in diameter. In an average piece of printing, there are some 15,000 dots per square centimeter. Such printing cannot be even slightly out of register. Toppan prides itself on having the finest technology anywhere in the ultra-minute micro-world in its platemaking. Further developing that precision logically leads to the production of photomasks for ICs and LSIs. Moreover, throughout the manufacture of precision electronic components, which use photo-processing technology as the base for ultra-minute processing, the latest electronics technology is applied. Photomasks are inspected for measurement using laser beams. In fact, it is a printing company's wide range of technological expertise in such fields as ultra-high-level photoengraving technology, chemistry, optics, physics, industrial machinery, electronics and engineering that makes the production of precision electronic components possible.

Toppan's Long-Term Strategy

It has been often said in Japan that Toppan is a mirror of Japan's GNP. The firm is closely involved with a wide range of customers whose needs change. The printing industry has an inseparable relation with the movement of the society and economy, and this industry must meet changing requirements in the outside world. The pace of changing conditions is, in fact, intensifying. Long-term strategic planning is therefore increasingly critical. Toppan's determination of strategy is based on the following considerations:

- Lessons and forecasting based on past experience;
- Exact analysis and judgment based on social conditions;
- Taking the best advantage of Toppan's strengths;
- Crisis control and contingencies in the event that the forecasts are incorrect; and
- Appropriate timing.

In addition, Toppan is mindful of the following items related to strategic implementation:

- To make all preparations in advance;
- To support rapid decision-making with relevant information and appropriate organizational structures;
- To run an appropriate portfolio of business activities;
- To concentrate on human resources and funds;
- To continually refine conventional printing processes;
- To achieve in-house agreement on strategy;
- To promote individuals of talent;
- To encourage an in-house entrepreneurial spirit; and
- To demand high quality throughout the firm.

Technology will continue to play a key role in Toppan's long-term strategy. Toppan maintains one central research laboratory, the Central Research Center, and three other research laboratories, divisional research and development departments, which serve each business division, and an Information Processing Systems Center.

The Central Research Center is mainly engaged in fundamental and applied research with a view toward expanding the application of printing techniques. The other three research laboratories and the divisional R&D departments are involved in the research and development of the products of the divisions concerned. Costs directly related to the operation of these laboratories for the four fiscal years ended May 31, 1984, were ¥1.430 million ($6.356 thousand); ¥1.630 million ($7.244 thousand); ¥1.840 million ($8.178 thousand); and ¥2.200 million ($9.778 thousand), respectively.

This R&D activity has already led to significant achievements, particularly from its extensive research in electronics. Indeed, Toppan intends to concentrate on electronic and computer technology, and to combine such technology with other work in its research and development laboratories and departments. For example, Toppan has applied electronic and computer technology to such tasks as typesetting, plate-making, printing, binding and many kinds of finishing, creating an extensive line of machinery and processes that are marketed in Japan and exported.

Toppan has also actively developed precision electronic components production technologies. As integrated circuits, such as LSIs and VLSIs, have increased their capacities from 16 kilobits and 64 kilobits to 256 kilobits and one megabit, Toppan has developed software for circuit design technology to produce photomasks, production technology for video-camera color filters, and high-resolution shadowmasks for CRT terminals. Toppan is also currently developing solid-state video-camera color filters.

Toppan was the first company in Japan to develop IC cards with built-in integrated circuits for use as credit cards and medical record cards, as well as in industrial applications. IC cards are at the heart of Toppan's industrial strategy to act as an interface between precision electronics and information communications.

Toppan is also developing advanced packaging materials and concepts to meet the constantly changing requirements of its customers, especially in the food, pharmaceuticals and electronics fields.

The company is now moving toward the development of a new information system, linking computers and new telecommunications technology with printing. The firm is tackling this task from both marketing and technological perspectives. In June 1983, Toppan established its Information Processing Systems Center. This center develops and offers software based mainly on Toppan's development of characters and images for various types of services, including home shopping, home banking, data reference, information control of commodity distribution, and optical publications. Many of these services will soon use new technologies, including communications satellites; cable media, such as VRS (video response system) or CATV (cable television); and storage media, such as the laser discs. This center develops various information systems, such as the digital communications system, which connects customers and Toppan for market research, new product development, and sales activities.

In the area of marketing, Toppan is helping to develop home shopping, home banking, and various data retrieval services, distribution information control, electronic publishing and others. Toppan is now planning to emerge as a software house by developing software based on characters and information processing. Toppan believes that—in the 21st century—not only Japan, but the entire world will become a total network through computers and communications technology.

In Japan, developments in electronics technology and in the field of information systems are expected to lead to a broad network throughout the country of interconnecting computers and digital communications. The Japanese Government is promoting an information network system plan (INS) by which a digital communication network made of optic fibers will cover Japan toward the end of this century. Both the public and the private sectors are now working hard on developing businesses related to INS.

In anticipation of the approaching 21st century, Toppan is in active pursuit of a fusion of printing, computers, and electronic communications from every vantage point, as seen in Figure 5. The firm aims to be well positioned by virtue of its experience in printing and electronics, and because of its determined strategy to be at the leading edge of these technologies.

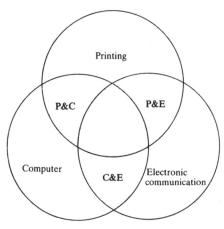

FIGURE 5. The three technologies.

Epilogue

Since its establishment in 1900, Toppan's expanding strategy has been to move perpendicularly from upstream to downstream, and horizontally into many related fields, like precision electronic components, which still have printing technologies as their core. Such expansion was encouraged by the following forces:

- Society's changing demands for the printing industry;
- The close linkage of printing companies with the broad movements of society and the economy;
- The requirement that the printing industry have a wide and close relationship with other industries and with the community; and
- Close cooperation with customers in meeting their needs since the printing industry must rely on orders from these same customers to exist and prosper.

In this environment, Toppan has thus far made strategic choices based on its past experience, on its assessment of options in view of its limited resources (human resources, materials, funds and technology), and on the vast opportunities available. The result is the amoeba-like strategy of diversification.

Mr. Suzuki, President of Toppan, phrases a slogan every year at the beginning of the year, and these slogans represent the company's strategy. The most recent slogans were:

"Let's become individuals of inter-businesses to the bottom."
"Offense is the best defense."
"Let's devote ourselves to basis and spearhead."

The latest slogan, in 1985, was:

"Let's all master printronics,"

amalgamating two words, printing and electronics. Perhaps the key overall word for characterizing Toppan is "interface." Toppan helps publishing companies in planning and editing. For consumer firms, Toppan takes charge of market research and the designing of packages and promotional materials. Thus, in Japan, integrated printing companies are suppliers of information in a broad sense. Toppan has made its particular declaration of "& industry." "&" is just what symbolizes Toppan; it means combination and harmony. The firm does nothing other than act as an "interface." That is Toppan's consistent strategic policy, as well as the foundation for Toppan's technology strategy.

New Approaches for the
Strategic Management of Technology

Graham R. Mitchell

ABSTRACT. *Technology is an increasingly important element in the business of many large corporations; its impact, however, is complex and often difficult to integrate into the strategic management process. This difficulty arises in part because technical advances — in addition to providing new ways to implement existing business strategy — often bring about the need to rethink that strategy. Not only does this imply that business management has to accept a wide role for the technologist in the formulation of strategy, but also that technical management must broaden its approach beyond the traditional focus on the direction of projects, and begin to address the* strategic management of technology. *New conceptual approaches may be needed to accomplish this, and this paper discusses the implementation of one such approach for the planning of technology in a major corporation, and its extension to the determination of strategy for the corporate laboratory.*

Scientists and engineers, not unnaturally, often consider the growth of scientific knowledge to be the basis of human progress. The general public frequently has a less exalted view of the role played by science and technology. These fundamentally different perceptions are brought into sharp focus in many modern industrial corporations where the general management community — which is strongly influenced by financial, legal and other business disciplines — tends to regard technology and enginering as just another contributing function within the business. In this view, the role of the engineer is primarily to carry out those programs which are needed to implement the strategies developed by business management. While recognizing the importance of markets, however, within its own ranks the technical community may well regard achievements by its peers around the world, and overall global technical trends as a far more reliable guide to technical and, hence, business opportunity than the formally documented strategies prepared by others within the corporation.

At the present time, a number of environmental trends throughout a wide range of businesses are leading both general and technical management to the conclusion that the strategic importance of technology is increasing. These two communities, however, still often experience difficulty in reaching agreement on priorities within

Graham R. Mitchell is Director of Planning for GTE Laboratories Incorporated, where his responsibilities have included the development of the strategic planning process for the central laboratories and technology planning for the corporation.

the corporate technical program, as their respective traditional analyses and perspectives of their respective disciplines frequently tend to polarize the discussion.

It is sometimes argued that the satisfactory resolution of the issues of technical strategy must await the emergence of a generation of general managers who are equally at home with issues of technology, or—alternatively—for R&D managers totally comfortable in the multiple aspects of the business world. This paper suggests that there are alternative solutions, short of wholesale conversion or long-term re-education of the principal protagonists. It is suggested that the best practical approach to this problem involves the creation and application of a framework which integrates the seemingly conflicting viewpoints. The framework allows both communities to discuss the trade-offs between short- vs. long-term perspectives and between evolutionary and revolutionary alternatives, as well as channeling technical resources to appropriate priorities on a mutually acceptable basis.

Issues for General Management

Many of the more attractive business areas in the United States—as measured in terms of potential growth or profitability—are subject to rapid technological change and technical obsolescence. Even in less rapidly growing business areas, continued research and development, as well as investment in leading-edge technologies, are often necessary for survival. Senior general management throughout US industry is repeatedly faced with the need to make resource allocations for technology to accomplish a wide range of strategic purposes. Whether trained as technologists or not, the challenge to general management can be daunting.

In many different industries, general managers are recognizing that these technical trends are changing the rules of business. For example, the rapid rate of advance of microelectronics is shortening the life of many products throughout a wide range of markets. Even the boundaries between hitherto distinct market segments are becoming blurred as the result of technical change. This is occurring between telecommunications and computing. General management's task is particularly difficult where the corporation's businesses are driven by rapid advances in a number of technical fields, or when a fast-moving technology underlies several different product lines or services.

Issues for Technical Management

Many of these same trends raise a complementary set of questions for technical management. A wide appreciation by the corporation of the growing importance of technology may not necessarily be seen by the R&D manager as a total blessing. He will almost certainly be quizzed more frequently on the business relevance of his programs, and be asked to define more clearly the linkage between the technical programs under his control and the business strategy. In addition, he will probably be required to participate more actively in the formulation of business strategy, for example, by characterizing technical trends and by providing assessments of the technical strength of the corporation's major competitors.

In the present environment, he is also likely to be experiencing a combination of global pressures which create a significant tension in his portfolio of programs, and tend to drive technical resource allocation in opposing directions at the same time. On one hand, the general explosion of scientific and technical activity in academic, industrial and government centers throughout the world is helping to create many new technical fields. These trends force R&D management to consider an expanding range of alternatives and a *broader* array of technologies within the R&D program. On the other hand, competitors operating from a large base in global markets may develop greater *depth* or expertise in key technical areas. This pressures management to *focus* resources to try to gain greater capability in the narrower range of technologies most critical to the survival of the business. If the total level of available technical resources is fixed, the dilemma can be illustrated by Figure 1. The explosion in science and technology can be seen to force decisions up the curve, while the global concentration of markets tends to force them down.

Need for an Integrated Framework

As a first step towards action, business and technical management need to agree on a common set of priorities.[1]

Often, the issue which is ultimately the most frustrating and difficult to resolve in the industrial setting concerns the degree to which technical programs should be targeted merely to the support of the existing strategies for the business, as opposed to providing opportunities for significant and sometimes revolutionary change.

The underlying positions in the discussion are often deeply rooted in education and professional experience. Usually the business view is that technology and engineering are best thought of as a functional capability, vying for resources with marketing, manufacturing, operations and other elements of the organization. In

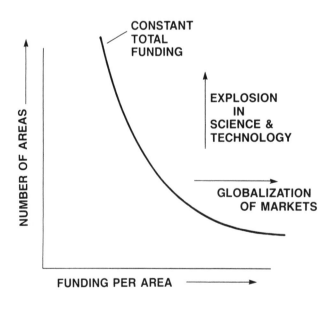

FIGURE 1. **Strategic Pressures on Technical Resources**

this view, technology is perceived as a subset of business. To the young technologist, however, business is often perceived as a subset of the general "technological ascent of man," as indicated in Figure 2.

The principal strategic challenge in the management and planning of technical programs within industry is thus to capitalize on and integrate these two seemingly contradictory viewpoints. What is needed is a framework which guides technical resource allocation to an appropriate balance between these two perspectives.

The implementation of this framework poses challenges to both communities. For business management, it requires acceptance of an enlarged role for the technologist in the formulation of business goals and strategy. For technical management, it implies that the traditional focus on the *management of projects* be extended to include a greater emphasis on the strategically more important issue of the *management of technology*.

Framework for Technology Management

Creation of a Common Language

The first step in communicating the impact which technology is expected to have on the business of the corporation and in managing the distribution of strategic resources is to set up a common language.

When defining "technologies," scientists and engineers are likely to speak in terms of skills or disciplines, such as solid state physics, circuit design, or heat transfer. The general business community—and for that matter the public at large—is more likely to speak in terms of classes of products, such as integrated circuits, computers or—even more broadly—as communications systems. These differences are not simply semantic, but indicate contrasting perceptions as to what is most significant. The technologist's definition deals with *input*, that is, the skills needed to build the product or service. The general manager's definition focuses on the *output*, the actual product or service, often with some sense of where or what the impact might be.

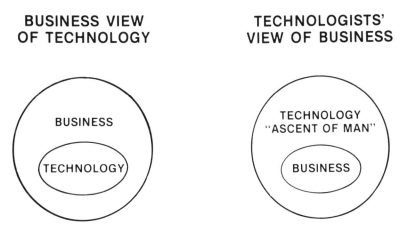

BUSINESS VIEW
OF TECHNOLOGY

TECHNOLOGISTS'
VIEW OF BUSINESS

BUSINESS

TECHNOLOGY

TECHNOLOGY
"ASCENT OF MAN"

BUSINESS

FIGURE 2.

Various taxonomies have been proposed for the characterization of technical effort.[2] In my view, the most effective approach, which communicates to both communities and clarifies the impact and relevance of technology to the business, is to *combine* the technical skills and their applications in a common definition. Specific terminology varies among organizations, but this unit of analysis is often called the "Strategic Technical Area" (STA), and its definition includes four components: 1. The skills or discipline → 2. which are applied to → 3. a particular product or service → 4. which addresses a specific market need.

An example of an STA definition that covers *Integrated Circuit Processing* is:

"1. The principal skills include lithographic techniques (photo, x-ray, electron beam) for defining fine geometries on semiconductors, as well as high-temperature solid state chemistry and thin film processing. 2. These are applied to the fabrication of semiconductor integrated circuits, 3. which are used in a wide range of switching and transmission products 4. throughout the telecommunications industry."

Identifying STAs — Building the Network

The underlying situation which gives particular value to the STA is that, in many large industrial corporations, similar technical skills and expertise are widely applicable to product or service areas in different parts of the organization. In many corporations, there is a *de facto network* of technical expertise, which often cuts across to the formal management and organization structure. While this linkage and synergy may be understood by the technical specialists, it is unlikely to be widely recognized at all management levels. This network provides insight and power to drive the businesses in new technical directions, some of which may challenge the conventional wisdom as articulated by the formal business plans.

The simplest way to start defining the STA is at the operating unit level (strategic business unit) with the array of product lines or services which it produces. For each of these product lines or services, the engineers and scientists are challenged to identify the critical skills necessary to maintain strong or leadership positions in the business. The number of STAs developed per product line or service depends on the complexity of the product or service. Usually three or four technical areas, however, are enough to identify the most critical skills.

As the exercise is repeated for adjacent products or services, it becomes clear that many of the same underlying strengths or skills may be utilized. Thus, definitions can be enlarged, broadened and an STA/product line (or service) matrix can be developed as shown in Figure 3. This illustrates that the underlying skill in, for example, the design of high-density integrated circuits or software engineering may be recognized as critical in several adjacent product lines.

As the process is extended to all business units across the corporation, numerous instances of parallel technical expertise will usually emerge. STAs originally developed for each product or service line may be broadened, and business unit, divisional, group and eventually corporate-level STAs may be defined. Somewhere in the region of 15 to 20 STAs seems optimum for analysis at each organizational level.

The perspective addressed by STAs automatically broadens as they are aggregated

Strategic Technical Area (STA)	Product Line 1	Product Line 2	Product Line 3	Etc.
Integrated Circuit Fabrication	X			
Integrated Circuit Design	X	X	X	
System Architecture		X		
Software Engineering	X	X	X	

FIGURE 3. STA/Product Line Matrix for a Telecommunications Product Business Unit

to a higher organizational level. At the lowest level of aggregation, the time horizon is shortest, the critical technical issues most immediate, and the coupling to business goals most direct. At the division and group level, this perspective lengthens. In the final aggregation at the corporate level, appropriate broad strategic issues, such as the provision of long-term technical strength and broad technical human resource requirements for the corporation for the next five years or longer, emerge directly from the identification of overall corporate technical needs by means of the STA analysis.

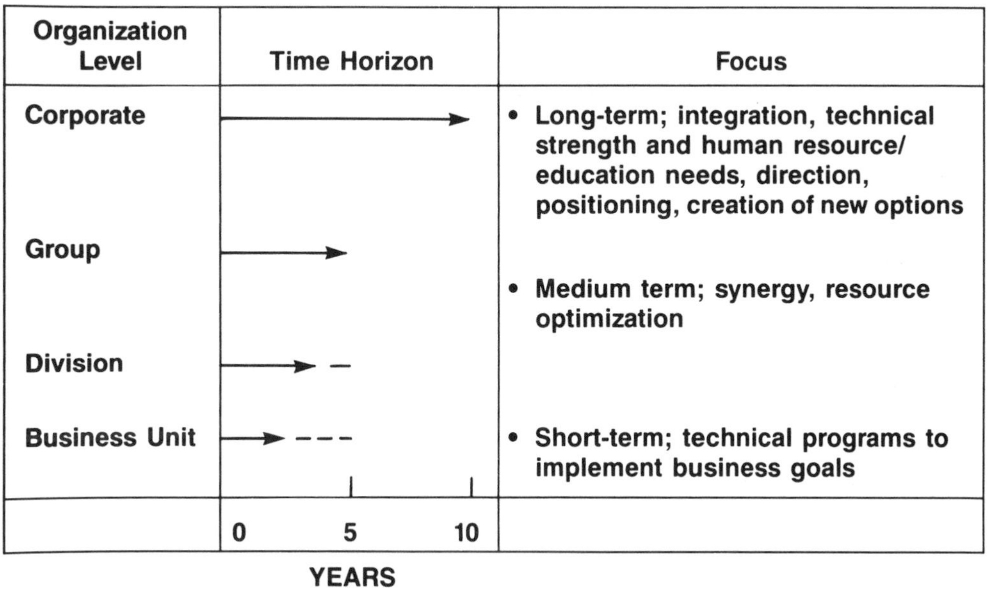

Organization Level	Time Horizon	Focus
Corporate	⟶	• Long-term; integration, technical strength and human resource/ education needs, direction, positioning, creation of new options
Group	⟶	• Medium term; synergy, resource optimization
Division	⟶ –	
Business Unit	⟶ – – –	• Short-term; technical programs to implement business goals
	0 5 10	

YEARS

FIGURE 4. STA Perspective at Different Organization Levels

Resource Allocation by STA

STAs have been defined to include those technical skills most critical to the survival and growth of the corporation. These are also the target of the corporation's discretionary technical expenditures, *viz*, the R&D program. It is thus a relatively straightforward process to characterize the R&D program by STA, and to arrive at the present and planned resource allocation by STA. With the resource allocation included, the STA business chart takes on added power. The Xs in Figure 3 may be replaced by present and future resource commitments at all levels within the corporation, and the full companywide commitment to particular technical areas becomes clear for the first time.

At the very highest level of aggregation, it is usually possible to cluster the STAs into generic technologies, such as software, materials, electronics, etc. At this level, the matrix illustrates the degree to which the future of the corporation's businesses—in this case, GTE—are linked to those underlying technologies. The matrix shown in Figure 5, makes clear that the decision to participate in many of the most attractive markets implies a sustained and deep commitment to the underlying technology.

Managing Technology with the STA/Business Matrix

Dual Perspectives

The STA/product line, service, or business matrix, such as is seen in Figure 3, provides the framework needed to integrate the conflicting approaches to technical strategy.

A review of the distribution of technical effort *vertically*—that is, by product line or organization—deals directly with the general management question: "Is the

Generic Technologies	Business Areas		
	Telecommunication Services	Telecommunication Products	Electrical Products
Software	H	H	L
Telecommunication Systems	H	H	L
Electronics	M	H	M
Materials	L	M	H

KEY:

  Relative Coupling
    H = High
    M = Medium
    L = Low

FIGURE 5. Coupling to Generic Technologies

technical strategy viable, and to what extent is the distribution of technical resources consistent with the stated strategy of the business?"

A *horizontal* view through the matrix begins to answer the technical managers' question: "Where are the greatest technical opportunities for the corporation?" The horizontal view defines those technical areas which are most important to the corporation in aggregate and, at the same time, identifies the specific present and future business lines which will be most affected by advances in the underlying technology.

Vertical Analysis — Evaluation of Competitive Technical Strength

Assuming that the business objectives and strategy have been developed with sufficient precision to define *where* it is we wish to go, the first question to be addressed is, "Will the planned technical resource allocations get us there?" The answer depends very much on where we start competitively, and this raises the immediate question, "How good are we, compared with our major competitors?"

The STA has been defined as the technology most critical to the success of the business, and is hence the natural unit against which to compare competitors' technical strengths.

Comparisons should be made against the leaders in the field, and should combine internal and external assessments. A simple profile that indicates the number of technical areas, in which the business unit is behind, equal or leading, very graphically communicates to general management the technical health of the business. For example, groups with profiles shown in Figure 6A are reasonably healthy insofar as their competitive position is at least equal to the major competitors in over 70% of the technical areas most critical to the success of the business. The key issue is, of course, future trends. If projections show a deterioration in position, significant additional funding or alternative sources of technology may be required.

Those businesses which are technically very strong will have a profile such as the one shown in Figure 6B, and here the strategic question most frequently asked is, "Are the businesses effectively using this technical capability to expand position and exploit their full technical potential in the market?"

Businesses with the characteristic shown in Figure 6C clearly face questions of viability over the long haul. This profile may be either symptomatic of a business in poor health, or a principal cause of its future decline. In either case, this profile is a good indicator of the need for fairly drastic managerial action.

Horizontal Analysis — Technical Opportunities

A horizontal slice through the matrix identifies the multiple impact of a given technology throughout the various businesses of the corporation. The STAs, singly and in clusters, thus define precisely the technologies which are perceived to have the greatest effect on the future of the business. These are the areas for which technology forecasts, scenarios and projections are critical, and for which rapid technical advances are most likely to lead business strategy in new directions. For the profile

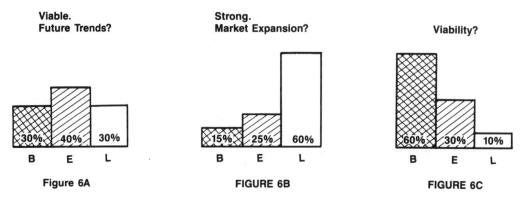

Percentage of technical areas most critical to the business where internal capability is

Behind   (B),
Equal to   (E), or
Leading   (L)

the principal competitors.

FIGURE 6. Competitive Technical Position

shown in Figure 5, detailed forecasts are required in key areas of software, electronics, telecommunication systems and materials.

Within the industrial setting, the ultimate purpose of developing a view of the future is to provide basis for action. In this context, it is more useful to discuss the uncertainty inherent in future projections in terms of timing. A prediction such as "In 1988 we expect the state of the art to be between 10^7 and 10^8 components on a chip" is likely to provoke very little response within the business community. If the uncertainty is stated in terms of timing, however, that is, "We expect 10^7 components on a chip to be available between 1987 and 1989," we can then force the question, "What implications does this have for the business, and what should we do in response?" The major uncertainty that remains to be discussed is *when* will it be appropriate to do it.

From an operational standpoint, the horizontal analysis identifies similar pockets of competence within large organizations and in this way develops the networks which are essential to technical information transfer throughout the corporation. Strengths in one area can be used to bolster and lead the development of technology in another, and thus promote synergy between operations.

Alignment of Technical and Business Strategy

Technical strategy may be most easily discussed and related to business strategy by answering two questions:

● Where is it we wish to go?
● How (technically) do we intend to get there?

It is often useful to define the first question in terms of the overall market strategy we wish to accomplish. Market strategies can be classified as *defending* present positions in the market, *extending* them, or developing *new* markets. Technical programs are targeted to these market strategies, and the resources can be characterized appropriately.

In addressing the second question as to *how* technically to achieve the desired impact on markets, the underlying technical strategy is determined by the present state of knowledge within the organization.

- If the technical challenge can be addressed through techniques, skills and expertise already well developed and resident in the organization, then the issues of strategy are reduced to the provision of adequate resources for the program.
- Alternatively, if the required technical expertise is available to leading competitors, but not resident in-house, the preferred technical strategy may include joint ventures, joint programs and licensing.
- On other occasions, when the required knowledge is neither available in-house nor available from external sources, R&D programs targeted toward *innovation* may be required.

The distribution of technical programs and effort can be arrayed to illustrate this combination of market and technical strategy. The variation in the distribution of resources within the matrix that occurs between individual business units is usually significant, and reflects both differences in business strategy and the varying sensitivity of different business lines to technology.

Figure 7A illustrates a stable business with mature product lines; Figure 7B illustrates a business unit adapting a competitor's technology; and Figure 7C illustrates a research laboratory in which program objectives incorporate more market and technical risk.

Strategy for a Corporate Laboratory

Technical Strategy

These approaches have been applied throughout GTE, and have been particularly useful in developing strategy for the central laboratory.

GTE, in common with many of its industrial peers, operates a corporate laboratory to provide support and leadership to the technical organizations of the business operations. Its mission includes leadership in areas of technology critical to the corporation and areas beyond the historic scope of the business.

The experience of major US corporations suggests that the development of strategy, as well as coupling and technology transfer to operations, is a complex issue for this kind of laboratory and requires continuous attention. The companywide STA/business matrix can be of major value in clarifying the strategy for the corporate laboratory. It identifies those areas in which the corporation's technical strengths and present programs are concentrated and, through the "horizontal" analysis, suggests where technical opportunity is greatest. Because the central laboratory

MARKET STRATEGY

DEFEND — Hold on, or catch up in existing Market

EXTEND — Major share growth and participation in adjacent segment

NEW — Growth beyond present Markets and Diversifications

TECHNICAL STRATEGY

EVOLUTIONARY — Application of known technology (existing internal capability)

COMPETITOR — Application of competitor's technical approach

INNOVATION — Development of exploitation of the inventions of a basic new technical approach

TECHNOLOGY / MARKET

	DEFEND	EXTEND	NEW
EVOLUTIONARY	60		
COMPETITOR		10	10
INNOVATION			10

RISK ⟶

FIGURE 7A

	DEFEND	EXTEND	NEW
EVOLUTIONARY	10		
COMPETITOR	25	65	
INNOVATION			

RISK ⟶

FIGURE 7B

	DEFEND	EXTEND	NEW
EVOLUTIONARY	5		
COMPETITOR	5	20	20
INNOVATION	10	25	25

RISK ⟶

FIGURE 7C

FIGURE 7.

programs are designed to complement and lead the technical activities of operations, priorities will include a significant number of the more attractive and unaddressed opportunities illustrated by the matrix.

STAs for a Corporate Laboratory

Operationally, the technical work of the GTE research laboratory is managed and budgeted through more than 100 individual projects. Discussion of the overall corporate technical strategy can be tortuous and frustrating, if it is approached at this level of detail. The STA is the appropriate unit for discussion of strategy, because many projects can be grouped within a single STA, and funding projections may be developed for a number of years. Dealing with the STA quite naturally forces the R&D community—at all levels of the organization—to move from operational issues and address strategy. It is one thing to ask for funding for a one-year project, and quite a different experience to face a senior audience requesting 20 times this amount for each of the next five years.

Developing a Consensus

While the detailed process for deriving technical priorities is analytical and based on the potential contribution the program can make to the corporation, at the highest level of management the process is partially judgmental and political. The STAs are valuable in achieving a consensus at this level. The leaders of various business groups can be asked to rank the laboratory STAs in order of priority. The process, as well as clarifying the needs of the various organizations and indicating an overall aggregate priority, tends to communicate the diversity of the different constituencies within the corporation.

Some STAs are built from traditional strengths within the laboratory, and the technical capability in the area is—by world standards—very high. In other areas, the historic strengths may have been relatively low, and the present capability is still being developed. If this assessment of STA technical strength is plotted against the overall STA priority, the top left of the chart illustrates those areas where high priority within the company is matched by the greatest technical strength in the laboratory. It is clear that the greatest pressure for improvement (and additional resources) will be directed to those areas of lower capability where the overall need is perceived to be the highest, *i.e.*, the bottom left of the chart.

Newly introduced technical areas make their first appearance at the bottom right of the chart. With technical success and recognition by operations, they move toward the top left. The path taken will vary. Scientific advances will usually bring a vertical movement as the work achieves peer recognition within the technical community before it moves across the chart into operations. This is shown by Path A, and might typically describe exploratory work on new materials unfamiliar to operations. Occasionally, there is a great deal of market pull for a newly emerging technical area, and this is illustrated in Path B. This has occurred in many laboratories with expert systems or, more generally, with artificial intelligence, where government interest and exposure in the technical and general press has stimulated interest in these nontraditional software areas.

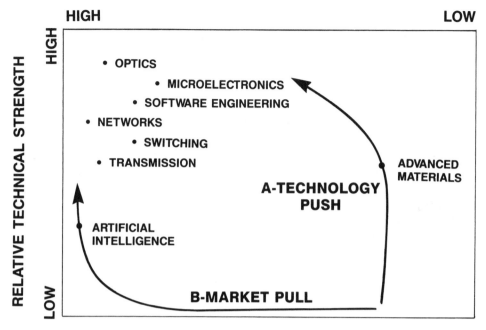

FIGURE 8. Relative Priority

Conclusions

This structure has taken several years to build, and has required continuing modi-
fication and refinement. While it is recognized as only one of the tools needed in
the *management of technology*, it has achieved one of its major purposes: It does
provide a common language for the discussion of technical priority and strategic
funding at all levels from the laboratory staff to the highest management within
the corporation. It forms the backbone of the strategic planning system for the corporate laboratory, and underpins the company-wide technology planning system,
which identifies major strategic technical issues at all levels within the corporation.

Notes

1. A broad treatment of this topic is given in Lowell W. Steele, *Innovation in Big Business* (New York: American
   Elsevier Publishing Co., Inc., 1975).
2. Additional discussions of the use of strategic technical areas in the determination of technical strategy are given
   in Domenic Bitondo, "Linking Technological and Business Planning," *Research Management*, November
   1981); and in Domenic Bitondo, "Technology Planning in Industry—The Classical Approach," Chapter 11, in
   Milan J. Dluhy and Kan Chen, eds., *Planning and Interdisciplinary Perspectives* (in press).

The Status of Technology Strategy in Europe

Pedro Nueno and Jan P. Oosterveld

ABSTRACT. This paper describes a new model of technology strategy that is implemented by European institutions. Focusing with some detail on the examples of the Research and Development programs of the European Economic Community in the areas of electronics and biotechnology, the pecularities of this model are analyzed. One of the characteristics of this model is the establishment of many R&D-related linkages between companies, research institutions, and governments at the regional, national and international levels. The evolution of this model and its success will be associated with factors such as the type of leadership required by this multidimensional process, the extent to which European organizations learn to manage the many linkages and develop the managerial capabilities needed to make progress in this linked cooperative project, and the ability to share the results of the cooperative effort combining competition and cooperation.

A new model of technology strategy formulation and implementation is emerging in Europe. Primarily, but not exclusively, under the leadership of the European Economic Community, this model emphasizes the establishment of various types of links between companies and institutions, both government-owned and private, at the national and international levels. European companies realize that only a linked model can give them access to technologies for which successful development might be beyond the capabilities of a single company. Also, Europe offers an open market where both American and Japanese companies have been operating for years, thus making easier the establishment of linkages between European and US or Japanese firms.

The model includes mechanisms for the development of technological forecasts and for the organization of the implementation of coordinated R&D in Europe. The structure of this process also takes into account all social stakeholders.

The remainder of this decade will be a critical period for European industry. If

Pedro Nueno is an industrial engineer and holds a doctorate in Business Administration from Harvard University. He is currently Professor of Management at the Instituto de Estudios Superiores de la Empresa at the University of Navarra in Barcelona, Spain. He is author of a number of books and articles on the management of technology and international business. Dr. Nueno is a member of the Board of the European Foundation for Management Development in Brussels.

Jan P. Oosterveld is an industrial engineer, and is at present Industrial Manager of Video Equipment at Philips International B.V. Eindhoven, The Netherlands. He has held management responsibilities at Philips in various countries. He attended the Eindhoven University of Technology, The Netherlands, and IESE at Navarra University.

this model of technology strategy succeeds, it can provide a framework for further economic integration and for a coordinated process of innovation where companies — big and small, government-owned and private, European and nonEuropean — could participate in building a tightly knit economic system that would help the old continent regain a competitive position in the world markets.

The Environment

Europe is experiencing problems that are associated with economic decline. Such is the perception of politicians, academics, industrialists, and social leaders in general. Reports, conferences, and the media all analyze the situation from different perspectives.[1] What was termed the energy crisis in the 1970s is termed the unemployment crisis in the 1980s. Table 1[2] shows data on the evolution of unemployment in Europe with the number of unemployed reaching 15 million within the European Economic Community alone in 1985.

Industrial production, productivity and trade have all performed poorly compared to Japan, as shown in Table 2.[3] The US and Japan have enjoyed a positive net balance between the creation and destruction of jobs, but this has not been the case in Europe.

Looking at the technology sector, it is also clear that Europe lags behind the United States and Japan. The indicators of technical superiority shown in Table 3[4] require no further comment. According to EEC studies[5], about 50% of the employed civilian workforce in the industrialized countries in 1980 was in "Information."

The information technology industry is expected to grow 8–10% per annum until 1990, reaching an overall turnover of $500 billion US (at 1980 prices) by that time. The EEC, however, despite having a trade surplus in information technologies in 1975, suffered a trade deficit of $5 billion in 1980, losing a share in its own market, which Community-based industry supplied to a mere 34%. In addition, an analysis of the trade deficit shows that the EEC primarily imports high technology products (such as central processing units) and exports products based on relatively mature electronic technology.

Table 1: Increase in number of registered unemployed in Europe

	FRG	FR	IT	NL	B	L	UK	IR	DK	GR	EUR-10
Additional unemployed (10^3)	1073	685	541	278	178	1	1680	57	144	42	4680
% increase relative to mid-79	122%	49%	33%	132%	53%	104%	121%	64%	105%	133%	68%
Level of unemployment at 1/82 (% of active population)	7.5	9.0	9.9	9.4	13.1	1.3	11.8	12.0	10.7	2.1	

Source: The Commission of the European Communities, Eurofutures

Table 2: Selected economic indicators

		France	W. Germany	Italy	UK	Japan
Share of World	1980	9.1	15.3	6.0	7.0	13.3
Trade Total %	1990	8.5	15.0	5.7	5.9	14.5
GDP Growth	1972/79	3.7	2.8	3.1	1.9	5.4
Rates	1980/90	3.0	2.3	2.7	1.3	4.7
Total Export	1975/80	6.1	5.9	6.2	1.3	9.5
Growth Rates (annual average)	1980/90	4.4	4.9	5.0	1.0	6.7
Productivity	1971/79	n.a.	0.29	0.28	0.14	0.42
Growth Rate (annual average)	1979/90	0.31	0.37	0.25	0.25	0.63
Employment in Manufacturing	1980	93.4	97.4	n.a.	93.3	94.9
Industry (Index 1975 = 100)	1990	91.3	104.0	n.a.	82.3	98.3
Car Exports as %	1975	13.4	22.8	6.8	4.5	1.4
of Total World	1980	13.7	16.1	6.2	1.0	22.9
Exports	1990	14.7	11.5	5.3	0.0	27.7

Source: Rainald V. Gizycki and Ingri Schubert, *Microelectronics: A Challenge for Europe's Industrial Survival.*

This gloomy environment has an influence on the types of reactions that are to be found in business, national and regional governments, and supranational institutions throughout Europe. There seems to be a consensus on the need to react quickly, to assign considerable resources, and to coordinate efforts, if European industry wishes to remain a relevant competitive force in the near future.

Table 3: Indicators of technological superiority

Indicator of Technological Superiority	Year	USA	W. Europe	Japan
Proportion of MOS Production	1980	41%	29%	38%
in Total Semiconductor Production	1985	57%	37%	55%
Proportion of Integrated Circuit	1980	77%	58%	62%
Production in Total Semiconductor Production	1985	87%	67%	77%
Degree of independence in	1980	154%	18%	86%
Integrated Circuit Production (Production/Consumption)	1985	177%	30%	100%

Technology and Strategy

Technology is society's pool of knowledge regarding the industrial arts[6]; technology is knowhow.[7] When technology becomes a key element in competition, it can be viewed as a critical resource that must be strategically managed. Technology and strategy have been studied as separate aspects.[8] Technology has been studied as an important variable in the areas of manufacturing management,[9] R&D management,[10] and management of international industrial deployment.[11] In the past decade, the recognition of the growing importance of technology has contributed to shortening the distance between the concepts of strategy and technology. Conceptually, technology has recently been considered by Abell as one of the three dimensions of business definitions (customer groups, customer functions, and technologies) versus the conventional two-dimensional concept of product-market strategy,[12] thus locating technology at the roots of the strategic planning process. Technology strategy is generally accepted as a component of the strategic management process into which it must be integrated, becoming a key issue in strategy formulation and implementation.[13]

Most models attempting to relate technology and strategy address the technology issue as one of the variables in the formulation of strategy in general, but the area of technology strategy has not been thoroughly researched. Some approaches to the formulation of technology strategy segment products and processes into their elementary technologies; it might even be possible to segment future (as yet unknown) products and processes into some of their component technologies (for instance, a future home-learning aid, currently neither available nor designed, will probably involve technologies such as voice recognition and friendly communication). These elementary technologies can then be handled with models derived from those available for strategy formulation in general. Matrix models—evolved, for instance, from the BCG matrices—represent technological importance on one axis and relative technology position on the other, producing a technology portfolio that can be the basis for technology strategy formulation.[14]

Horwitch suggests a different approach to integrating technology and strategic management.[15] As different modes of innovation (Mode I, entrepreneurial; Mode II, divisional; and Mode III, multi-institutional) become increasingly mixed and "linked" (through intraorganizational, domestic interorganizational, multinational interorganizational, and private-sector/public sector linkages), technological innovation requires strategic management from the top. Strategic management of technology then consists of giving the appropriate long-term direction to a variety of linkages in order to obtain the maximum benefit from the various innovation modes available in a complex international industrial setting. Hakansson and Laage-Hellman, along the same lines, also stress the concept of the firm as a network of technological and knowledge bonds that can be managed to develop a cooperative technology strategy.[16]

McGinnis and Ackelsberg point out that practicing managers have neglected the body of knowledge on managing innovation, managing change, technology transfer, and technology-related aspects in general.[17] This lack of assimilation that has prevented a better fit between technology and strategy is, in part, due to the fact that the available research in this area has never been synthesized in a way that could be applied in practice. They address the problem of improving innovation management and its relation to strategic planning with a framework based on the work of Burns and Stalker,[18] Daft and Becker,[19] Mohr,[20] Shepard,[21] and Utterback.[22]

As the business community becomes increasingly aware of the importance of integrating technology within the strategic management process, it develops a need for models and methodologies to implement this integration. Responding to this need, consulting firms (such as, for instance, Booz Allen and Hamilton and Arthur D. Little) have developed specific approaches to technology strategy formulation.

Technology Strategy in Europe

The area of technology strategy in Europe today is very complex. It could be analyzed from a variety of standpoints, which, for the purpose of simplicity will be reduced here to business level, government level (both national and regional), and European level (EEC and other supranational institutions).

Technology Strategy at the Business Level

At the business level, technology strategy has been handled by most European firms as a bottom-up process. In many firms, scientific and technical experts have been granted substantial powers of discretion in assigning priorities to R&D projects. The link between R&D and other areas of the business has been slight with some matters being of exclusive competence of R&D and the remainder being left to other areas of business management.

The level of integration achieved has generally been minimal. This serves to explain the paradox whereby notable successes in European research have nevertheless been notorious commercial failures in those businesses which financed their development. Commercial successes accompanied by success in technological innovation are the exception to the rule in Europe, and are most often found in firms which had achieved market domination in a given segment many years earlier, and which were able to maintain their positions, thanks to a continuous effort in product and process technology development. A good example of this is provided by the Philips Lighting Products Division, where continuous product leadership is allied to the development of the firm's own manufacturing equipment and a dominant market position inherited from previous years.

The management of those decisions affecting technology management (such as which technologies should be developed in-house, which should be acquired, what scope should be covered in specific areas, such as product, product-component-material-equipment) has also generally been relegated to the area of Technical Management within the firm. The separation of the technical and marketing departments into two powerful and, at times, antagonistic organizations, giving the firm a bicephalous structure, had frequently been encountered in European firms, even in those of small and medium size.

For many years, strategic planning focused on the marketing function with relatively little attention being paid to the search for industrial efficiency and even less to the technological aspect. This explains the modest nature of industrial concentration, despite the legal facilities which exist for its promotion within Europe. This reality has been borne out by the small number of mergers taking place, and the failure of certain attempts at concentration.

The failure of the Dutch Hoogovens and the German Hoesch merger in the steel industry illustrates this, as does the ill-fated Dutch-German alliance between Fokker and VWF in aviation, and contacts between Fiat and Citroën and Fiat and SEAT in the automobile industry, which failed to give birth to a company with relevant market share. The attempted merger between the British Dunlop and Italian Pirelli tire manufacturers, whose failure left Europe open to the Japanese, should also not be forgotten.[23] Moreover, in some of those situations where concentration did materialize (*e.g.*, Ciba-Geigy, Agfa-Gevaert, Philips-Grundig, etc.), this was not achieved without parallel structures being allowed to persist for long periods without the potential economies of scale — hoped for from concentration — materializing.

It was in the 1970s that the first efforts in search of industrial rationalization were seen. In some large firms, the process of strategic planning was geared towards simplification: fewer plants to manufacture the same product, simpler organizational structures, and disinvestment away from ventures unrelated to the central business.[24] Parallel to this, in small- and medium-sized businesses, greater stress was laid on the central business concept and productivity — with more superfluous activities being rooted out.

Strategic technology planning — from the top down — is a new phenomenon in many European businesses. It is beyond doubt that firms of a reasonable size possess staff qualified in strategic planning and aware of the need to formalize the process. In some large firms, a process of strategic technology planning has been carried out, but those responsible admit that such efforts have not been granted priority attention by top management, preventing their development beyond the stage of an interesting academic exercise. Along the same lines, it can be said that the leading consulting firms have not enjoyed great success in selling their services on technology strategy formulation projects within Europe.[25]

In the world of small business, technology is often handled with an entrepreneurial approach, also from the bottom up, with the difference that, in this case, the bottom is closer to the top. The company has certain technologies at its command, and, by using every conceivable means of packaging, handles the technologies in ways that they can be brought to the market. However, according to EEC studies, in Europe "the myth of the innovating small firm is firmly established but has little foundation in fact . . . apart from a rather unfavorable cultural background, the obstacles to the development of small firms are mainly financial (unsuitable capital market, lack of venture capital and a penalizing tax system)."[26]

The role of the small- and medium-sized companies in Europe, with regard to the development of technology, can only be seen in a linked fashion with large firms, because — on the one hand — about 50% of small firms in Europe are merely subcontractors, and — on the other hand — because the capital market is underdeveloped (access to venture capital is very limited, and over-the-counter-type mechanisms are either non-existent or just experimental).

Technology Strategy at the Government Level

In Europe it is important to take into account that technology strategy is a subject that is debated at both national-government level and at the level of regional governments within national states, giving rise to strategies at national and regional or local levels. These strategies find their expressions in laws, programs and proposals which tend to be binding on publicly owned firms and for those research centers dependent upon the public sector, while serving as guidelines for the private sector and in various bodies implementing the aforementioned regulations.[27] In several countries there exist systematized approaches, which attempt to influence the technology strategies of private companies by means of the state offering to participate in the risk-sharing, provided the project in question falls under a sector deemed to be of priority.[28] Magaziner shows how European nations have formulated industrial policies containing a technological component.[29] In the past few years, new elements of technology policy have been produced by national and regional governments.[30]

It is almost certain that, in most cases, the set of technology strategy measures adopted by national or regional governments would not survive a strategy evaluation test, and would appear to be little more than sets of measures that are not particularly internally consistent. It is also a generally held view that technology policies in European states are excessively geared to the short term, due to their links with the political process and ever-increasing financial limitations.[31] EEC member states spend an average of 1% of their GNP on public-sector-financed R&D. European governments do currently recognize the necessity to stimulate technological development. Most European governments are, however, in a paradoxical situation: On the one hand, the laying down of a series of social priorities has created rigidities in the economy (high public spending, the financing of which causes the "expulsion" of the private sector from the capital market, rigidities in labor legislation, high tax burdens), which discourage entrepreneurship and innovation, and, on the other hand, these same governments realize that only entrepreneurship and technological innovation can solve Europe's problems in the long term. This creates an ambiguous situation whereby incentives and disincentives for innovation exist side by side.

Technology Strategy at the European Supranational Level

Clearly, it is the technology policy of the European Economic Community which merits special attention here. Some Community officials would not accept the idea that the EEC already possesses a genuine technology strategy. The common research policy of the EEC was regulated until 1967 by the legal bases of the three communities: the European Coal and Steel Community, Euratom, and the EEC. The merger of the three communities in 1967 established the way toward coordinating research efforts carried out under different bodies. The oil crisis and the technological developments of the early 1970s led to the creation of a joint research development policy for the European Community as a "political unit." This founds its expression in the Council Resolution of January 14, 1974, on the coordination of national pol-

Table 4 – COMMUNITY, RESEARCH, DEVELOPMENT AND DEMONSTRATION ACTIVITIES

Activity	Code	Dur.	1982	1983	1984	1985	1986	1987	1988
1. AGRICULTURE AND FISHERIES									
Agriculture									
Agricultural Research	CSA, CONC	5 A	19.7 ME				8 ME		
Ligno-cellulosic Mat. for Animal Feeding	CONC	4 A					??? ME		
Fisheries									
Fisheries	CSA	4 A					5 ME		
2. INDUSTRY									
Industrial Technologies									
Community Bureau of Reference	CSA	5 A	10.3 ME			25 ME			
Nuclear Measurements and Reference Materials	JRC	4 A	48 ME			54 ME			
High Temperature Materials	JRC	4 A	16.6 ME			28 ME			
Basic Technological Research	CSA	4 A				135 ME			
Steel Research	ECSC	·	19 ME	17 ME					
Pilot /Demonstration Projects in Steel Industry	ECSC	·				50 ME			
Textile	CSA	3 A		3.9 ME					
Applications of New Technology	CSA	4 A				35 ME			
Foodstuffs 1	CONC	4 A			3.67 ME				
Foodstuffs 2	CONC	4 A	0.287 ME		0.78 ME				
Information Technologies									
Data Processing	CSA	7 A	25 ME			54 ME			
Microelectronics	CSA	4 A		40 ME					
Esprit	CSA			11.5 ME		48 ME			
Eurotra	CSA					16 ME			
Biotechnologies									
Biomolecular Engineering	CSA	4 A		15 ME					
3. TRANSPORT									
Aids to Coastal Navigation	CONC	3 A		2.1 ME					
4. RAW MATERIALS									
Raw Materials	CSA	4 A		54 ME					
5. ENERGY									
Nuclear Fission									
Reactor Safety	CSA	4 A	6.3 ME			31.8 ME			
Reactor Safety	JRC	4 A	174.5 ME			85 ME			
Reactor Development and Advanced Technologies	–	·	0.9 ME	1.1 ME					
Management and Storage of Radioactive Waste	CSA	5 A		43 ME					
Radioactive Waste Management	JRC	4 A	23.1 ME			47 ME			
Fissile Materials Control and Management	JRC	4 A	23.1 ME			44 ME			
Nuclear Fuel and Actinide Research	JRC	4 A	50.7 ME			55 ME			

Activity	Type	A	Values
Decommissioning of Nuclear Plants	CSA	5 A	4.7 ME / 12.1 ME
Utilization of HFR Reactor	JRC	4 A	54.5 ME / 59 ME
Fusion			
Controlled Thermonuclear Fusion – Gen. Prog.	CSA	5 A	301 ME
Fusion Technology	JRC		28.8 ME / 46.5 ME
Controlled Thermonuclear Fusion – JET	CSA		319 ME
Specific Credits for Projects of Eur. Significance	JRC	4 A	12.5 ME
Non-Nuclear Energies			
Energy (Developm. Renewable Sources – Rational Use)	CSA	4 A	105 ME / 379 ME
Solar Systems Testing Methods	JRC	4 A	25.5 ME / 22 ME
Habitat Energy Management	JRC	4 A	17 ME
Altern. Sources. Saving. Subst. of Hydrocarbons	DEMO	5 A	25 ME / 395 ME
Liquefaction and Gasification of Solid Fuels	DEMO	5 A	15 ME / 95 ME
Coal Research	ECSC	5 A	17 ME / 19.5 ME
6. DEVELOPMENT AID			
S/T for Development	CSA	4 A	40 ME
Indigenous S/T Research in Devel. Countries	CSA	4 A	60 ME
7. HEALTH AND SAFETY			
Radiation Protection	CSA	5 A	59 ME / 94 ME
Medical and Public Health Research	CONC	5 A	13.3 ME
Effects on Health of Workers Occ. Hazards	ECSC	5 A	9 ME
Ergonomics and Rehabilitation	ECSC	5 A	13 ME
Industrial Hygiene in Mines	ECSC	5 A	11 ME
Safety in Mining	ECSC	5 A	7 ME
Control of Pollution in the Iron and Steel Industry	ECSC	5 A	12.5 ME
Safety in Steel Industry	ECSC	2,5 A	15 ME / 1 ME
8. ENVIRONMENT			
Protection of the Environment	JRC	4 A	34 ME / 49 ME
Environment and Climatology	CSA. CONC.	5 A	42 ME / 12.5 ME
Application of Remote Sensing Techniques	JRC	4 A	18.5 ME / 29 ME
Industrial Risk	JRC	4 A	21 ME
Clean Technologies	DEMO	.	1.5 ME / 1.5 ME
Sea Protection		.	0.5 ME / 0.6 ME
9. IMPROVING EFFICACY OF S/T POTENTIAL			
Stimulation	—	2 A	7 ME
10. HORIZONTAL ACTIVITIES			
FAST	CSA	4,5 A	4.4 ME / 8.5 ME
Scientific and Technical Education and Training	CSA		8.8 ME
Utilization of R & D Results	—	.	1.3 ME / 1.95 ME
Programme Preparation and Evaluation	—	.	

icies and the definition of projects of interest to the Community in the field of science and technology.[32]

The EEC common research policy aims to enhance the effectiveness of research in member states by the selective use of available resources, and by concentrating on the most important sectors. It is geared toward medium- and long-term research and development. It takes into account the possibility of international cooperation, that is to say that small research groups, working in different locations, can still operate effectively as part of a larger research effort. The new scientific and technological knowledge generated by Community research can be used throughout the Community, thus contributing to European integration and strengthening Europe's potential as a worldwide competitor.[33] In May 1984, Community Research, Development and Demonstration Activities had an overall budget of 3300 million ECU (on April 13, 1985, the ECU was equivalent to 0.71 US dollars)[34] for the four years 1984–87 (see Table 4).

In 1978, the EEC set up a technology forecasting mechanism which was to serve as a key element for subsequent technology strategy formulation: the FAST (Forecasting and Assessment in the Field of Science and Technology) Program. The objective of FAST was to establish a long-term guidelines framework which could function as a basis for technology strategy formulation. The FAST Program tackled three major areas: a) Work and Employment, this being felt to be the most important potential program in the coming 10–15 years; b) the Information Society, since it was felt that the set of technologies related to electronics, information systems, and telecommunications were those which would have the greatest impact on the economy and society in general in the next 20 years, this making it vital that Europe be able to play a relevant role in these fields; and c) the Biosociety, since it was expected that biotechnologies would have a major impact on the world economy within the next 30 years.[35] Table 5 shows the eleven strategic issues identified by the FAST Program.[36]

The FAST Program can be considered as a general framework, which has given rise subsequently to a series of concrete strategic proposals in specific areas. The most important strategic projects are probably those which attempt to cover strategic issues corresponding to the Information Society and the Biosociety. The official *Journal of the European Communities* for November 26, 1983, published the "Proposal for a Council Decision," adopting the first European strategic program for research and development in information technologies (ESPRIT).[37] Table 6 shows the areas of R&D activity and infrastructure actions planned within ESPRIT. Table 7 shows the estimated resources needed to carry out the program at 9,268 manyears. Community estimates place the economic equivalent of these manyears at 1500 million ECU for the first five years (1984–88) or about 6% of the total industrial R&D investment in Information Technology in the EEC. The EEC plans to contribute 50% of this budget from its own resources, or 750 million ECU, the remaining 50% falling to European industry.

Similarly, in April 1984, the Commission of the European Communities presented a "Proposal for a Council Decision" to the EEC Council of Ministers for undertaking a multi-annual research action program of the European Economic Community in the field of biotechnology, covering the period from January 1985 to

Table 5: Strategic Issues Identified by the FAST Programme

The Strategic issues of Work and Employment	The Strategic issues of The Information Society	The Strategic issues of Bio-Society
—Renewal and Consolidation of the European Industrial Base	—Industrial Mastery of the New Information Technologies	—Foundation capabilities for European Bio-technology
—Mastering the Process of Technological Change	—The emergence of an International Information and Communication System	—Managing the Renewable Natural Resource System
	—Alienation or Active Participation by the Individual	—Biotechnology and Europe-Third World Relations
	—Creation of new jobs	—Health and Medical Research
	—Education Training and learning	

Source: Developed by the authors from the FAST documents (see (36))

Table 6: Areas of R & D activity and infrastructure actions planned within ESPRIT

1. Advanced microelectronics capability
   —computer-aided design, manufacture and test for very large-scale integrated circuits (VLSIC)
   —silicon IC process steps to 1-micron feature size
   —integration of process steps, leading towards computer-controlled VLSIC fabrication
   —process steps for submicron feature sizes in silicon and other semiconductor materials
   —techniques for interfacing ICs to their environment
   —research into optical information processing and transmission, notably integrated optoelectronics, optical switching and storage
   —novel information and image display technologies
   —novel organic and inorganic materials for electronics and optical technologies
2. Software technologies
   —scientific foundations
   —software development as an industrial activity
   —software development as an economic activity
3. Advanced information processing (AIP)
   —information and knowledge engineering, including expert systems
   —pattern recognition techniques and their application to interfaces with the environment, particularly intercommunication between human and machine
   —information and knowledge storage, including novel hardware technologies and advanced software techniques
   —computer architecture, particularly for parallel processing, leading to novel processing machines of advanced capability
   —design objectives and methods, of embedding trustworthy AIP concepts into VISIC

Table 6. (Continued)

4. Office systems
   — office systems science
   — office work-stations, document description languages, document creation and distribution man/machine interfaces
   — office communication systems including local area networks and their interconnection, integrated interactive text-voice-image-video communication and value-added functions
   — office filing and retrieval systems, easy access to and retrieval of knowledge
   — human factors, encompassing the interactions man/information handling systems
5. Computer integrated manufacture (CIM)
   — integrated system architecture for CIM systems
   — computer-aided design and engineering (CAD and CAE) systems of modular structure
   — modular computer-aided manufacture, test and repair systems and their integration with CAD, CAE
   — software and operating systems for assembly, robots, and numerically controlled machine-tools
   — imaging and control systems for the real-time capture and processing of 3D images and for generating appropriate responses, incorporating AIP techniques
   — VLSIC design and fabrication for CIM subsystems, sensors, etc.
   — demonstration models of CIM subsystems leading to complete CIM demonstrators for experiments in real life situations
6. Infrastructure actions
   — coordination of Community and Member States R & D, acquisition and dissemination of information within ESPRIT and from the world at large
   — coordination and documentation of standards within ESPRIT and their relationship with national and international standards
   — information exchange system (IES) to support good execution and management of R & D as well as appropriate dissemination of results.

Source: Commission of the European Communities. ESPRIT (see Note 37)

December 1989. In some aspects, this program was conceived as a parallel to the ESPRIT model. Table 8 shows the areas of R&D activity within the biotechnology program, and Table 9 the financial resources that would have to be drawn from the EEC budget.[38]

The initiative for technology strategy in Europe, however, does not emanate exclusively from the EEC. There exist other supranational institutions which also have a role to play in the process. One of these is known as COST, or European Cooperation in the Field of Scientific and Technical Research, which has been functioning for some 15 years.

COST has conceived with intentions similar to those underlying the EEC Council Resolution of January 14, 1974, in order to unify technology policies of the EEC. COST, however, includes all western European countries among its participants — 19 countries in total — not just EEC member states, although many of the R&D activities sponsored by COST are closely related to Community R&D. The emphasis of activities developed under COST is on the stimulation of cooperation at the

Table 7: Estimated resources needed to carry out the ESPRIT programme

ESPRIT PROGRAMME

Resource summary (man years)
Activities started during first phase (1984 to 1988)

	Pilot Projects 0	1984 1	1985 2	1986 3	1987 4	1988 5	1989 6	1990 7	1991 8	1992 9	1993 10	Total
Projects starting in year:												
0	230	325	327	192	125	30						999
1		420	551	629	540	519	20					2679
2			547	766	670	545	140					2668
3				328	428	450	256	68				1530
4					204	276	180	85	45			790
5						92	140	125	105	80	60	602
Total Man years	230	745	1425	1915	1967	1912	736	278	150	80	60	9268

Source: Commission of the European Communities. ESPRIT (see reference (37) p. 29)

Table 8. R & D activity within the proposed biotechnology program.

Action I. Research and Training
  Subprogram 1: contextual measures for R & D in biotechnology
    Measures to upgrade quality and capabilities of facilities, resources and support services
    — Bio-informatics
    — Collections of biotic materials
  Subprogram 2: Basic biotechnology
    Pre-competitive research and research through training in areas of basic biotechnology
    — Enzyme engineering
    — Genetic engineering
    — Physiology and genetics of species important to industry and to agriculture
    — Technology of cells and tissues cultured *in vitro*
    — Screening methods for the evaluation of the toxicological effects and of the biological
      activity of molecules
    — Assessment of risks
Other activities associated to other research programmes
    — Aquatic primary biomass (cost)
    — Plant in vitro culture (cost)
    — Involvement in the activities of the "Technology, growth and employment" working
      group created at the Versailles summit of 1982
Action II: Concertation
    A concertation activity addressed to improving standards and capabilities in the life
sciences and enhancing the strategic effectiveness with which these are applied to the social
and economic objectives of the EEC and its Member States.

Source: Commission of the European Communities COM (84) 230 final (38)

European level, the COST financing being limited. The R&D priority areas are in-
formatics, telecommunications, transport, oceanography, metallurgy and materials
science, environmental protection, meteorology, agriculture, food technology,
medical research, and health.[39]
  More recently, another supranational institution has come to the fore, reflecting
the concern of that part of European industry which is still in reasonably good health

**Table 9. Estimated expenditures associated to the
proposed biotechnology research program**

	Expenditures (Millions of ECU)
Action 1: Research and Training in Biotechnology	
— Subprogram 1: Contextual Measures for R & D	11.11
— Subprogram 2: Research and Training	69.00
— Actions associated to cost	1.50
— Participation in Versailles Working Party	0.50
Action II: Concertation	6.41
TOTAL	88.52

Source: Commission of the European Communities. COM(84)230 final (38)

Table 10. ROUNDTABLE OF EUROPEAN INDUSTRIALISTS MEMBERSHIP

Chairman:
Pehr G. GYLLENHAMMAR

V. Chairmen:
Umberto AGNELLI

Wisse DEKKER

Members:
Umberto AGNELLI, Deputy Chairman
FIAT SpA (ITALY)

Carlo De BENEDETTI,
   Chairman & Chief Executive Officer
OLIVETTI & Co (ITALY)

Sir John CLARK,
   Chairman & Chief Executive
THE PLESSEY COMPANY PLC (UK)

Wisse DEKKER, President
PHILIPS INDUSTRIES
   (THE NETHERLANDS)

Adolphe DEMEURE de LESPAUL,
   Chairman & Chief Executive Officer
PETROFINA S.A. (BELGIUM)

Sir Kenneth DURHAM, Chairman
UNILEVER PLC (UK)

Roger FAUROUX,
   Président Directeur Général
SAINT-GOBAIN (FRANCE)

Pehr G. GYLLENHAMMAR,
   Chairman & Chief Executive Officer
AB VOLVO (SWEDEN)

Bernard HANON,
   former Président Directeur Général
REGIE NATIONALE DES USINES
   RENAULT (FRANCE)

Karlheinz KASKE,
   President & Chief Executive Officer
SIEMENS AG (FRG)

Jean-Luc LAGARDERE,
   Président Directeur Général
MATRA (FRANCE)

Olivier LECERF,
   President Directeur Général
LAFARGE COPPEE (FRANCE)

Ian MACGREGOR,
   Chairman & Chief Executive
NATIONAL COAL BOARD (UK)

Helmut MAUCHER, Managing Director
NESTLÉ SA (SWITZERLAND)

Hans MERKLE,
   Chairman of the Supervisory Council
ROBERT BOSCH GmbH (FRG)

Curt NICOLIN, Chairman
ASEA AB (SWEDEN)

Antony PILKINGTON, Chairman
PILKINGTON BROTHERS PLC (UK)

Louis von PLANTA,
   Chairman & Managing Director
CIBA-GEIGY (SWITZERLAND)

Antoine RIBOUD,
   Président Directeur Général
BSN (FRANCE)

Stephan SCHMIDHEINY, Chairman
ETERNIT AG (SWITZERLAND)

Dieter SPETHMANN,
   Chairman of the Management Board
THYSSEN AG (FRG)

Jacopo VITTORELLI, Managing Director
PIRELLI SpA (ITALY / SWITZERLAND)

Source: Ray Eales "Europe's Industrialists revive the European Dream" *Multinational INFO*, Institute for Research and Information on Multinationals, Geneva, No. 7, February, 1985

as to the dangerous decline of Europe as a world competitor. The group in question is called the "Roundtable of European Industrialists," a list of whose members appears in Table 10. The group, under the leadership of Pehr Gyllenhammar, Chairman of Volvo, has met twice a year since April 1983 in an effort to launch projects that contribute to the revitalization and further integration of Europe.

   To promote high-technology firms, the group launched Euroventures BWBV, a venture capital company sponsored by Asea, Volvo, Fiat, Olivetti, Pirelli, BSN,

Lafarge Coppeé, Saint-Gobain, Philips and Bosch, which started operations in 1985. Euroventures will provide loans up to 15% of the equity of new high-technology businesses.[40]

The Roundtable also plans to become involved in major infrastructure and even education projects. Robert Bosch, the West German automobile components manufacturer, has submitted a plan to create a European Institute of Technology along the lines of the American MIT. In addition, the group has produced proposals with a total estimated budget of 60 million dollars for upgrading European infrastructure: the EuroRoute, a combination of bridge and tunnel (brunnel) that would connect the United Kingdom and France; Scandinavian road and rail links with the Continent; and a high-speed train network in Europe.[41]

A common characteristic of all these Community and extra-Community initiatives is that they have arisen as reactions to European decline, while they recognize the necessity to undertake supranational action coordinating all the resources Europe has at its disposal. They are intended to serve as a catalyst to direct technology strategy toward areas which are felt—either intuitively (Roundtable) or more formally (FAST)—to be of relevance for the future.

EEC technology programs take into account actions undertaken in member states (both public and private sectors thereof).[42] In this way, EEC programs complement and/or coordinate the activities of member states. At the same time, EEC policy is a useful reference framework for European states' strategies, both at the national and regional level, and the Community (such as the FAST Program) is used by ministries in different countries to formulate industrial and technology strategy.

The Process of Technology Strategy Formulation in the EEC

Perhaps more interesting are the framework and process by which technology policies come to be formulated in the EEC. At the same time, the learning process which appears to be taking place is worthy of specific attention, given its potential future consequences.

The process by which a community technology development program sees the light of day is complex, and does not follow a single pattern. Sometimes an idea occurs from the bottom up within the Commission and, after being formulated, is presented by the Commission to the Council of Ministers for the latter's approval. In these cases, the idea may have been the initiative of a Commission official, or it may have been transmitted to him from outside. The reverse process can also occur, whereby the idea originates in the Council of Ministers, who request the Commission to carry out a study and submit a proposal. In such a case, the idea could reach the Council via one of the ministers' own initiatives, or be the result of the interests of a specific industrial sector in a member state. The third path is that of the European Parliament, which can also generate ideas for the Commission, which, in turn, prepares a concrete proposal.

The drafting of Commission proposals is a deliberately open procedure, and experts and consultants of prestige external to the EEC are normally involved in the work. At the same time, a number of consultative bodies and advisory committees, which interact with the Commission (*e.g.*, CORDE, Committee on Research and

Development). These interactive bodies also fulfill the role of representing European businesses and trade unions.

Business representation is channeled through UNICE (the association of the European national employers organizations) and that of the trade unions through the ETUC (European Trade Union Confederation). A whole series of formal and informal contacts among Community officials responsible for drawing up proposals and the European environment take place around these consultative bodies. At the same time, exploratory contacts take place within the legislative bodies, Council and/or Parliament, to determine up to what point certain aspects can be included in the proposals tabled. An approved proposal, equipped with a budget and structure, provides a framework for the generation of technology; thus, it could be said that this is tantamount to a community technology strategy.

Once the framework has been established, a further complex process begins, namely implementation. A typical implementation model would consist of the tendering of proposals for the development of specific projects along the lines of objectives laid down in the framework. For the 1984 phase of the ESPRIT program, for instance, 441 proposals were presented, of which 90 were selected. Program management is also normally effected by a committee process. Thus, for example, ESPRIT is administered by the ESPRIT Management Committee, comprised of representatives of EEC member states, while this is counterbalanced by the ESPRIT Advisory Committee, in which industry and European research centers are included. These committees, supported by a jury of scientists of recognized international prestige, select the proposals to be approved. Obviously, scientific, political and economic criteria all have their say in this complex, if relatively open dynamic process.

The organization of meetings for the exchange of ideas is frequently a part of the implementation process. For example, in Autumn 1984, more than 600 people attended the first ESPRIT meeting held in Brussels. In these meetings, politicians, Community officials, scientists, academics and businessmen have the opportunity to exert individual or collectively organized influence on the evolution of the implementation process.

When dealing with technology strategy implementation, special consideration should be given to lobbies. Lobbying is carried out either directly by business appointing managers to this specific task, or indirectly via business organizations and specialized consulting firms. Some large firms devote considerable attention to this facet of management. This is particularly true in the area of electronics, information systems, and telecommunications, where a few large European firms have a huge amount of influence, allowing them to be more direct beneficiaries of EEC technology strategy. Community civil servants acknowledge the importance of this lobbying, which, in general, they value positively, since it contributes to closing the gap between the EEC and the European business world, as well as allowing for better understanding on the part of officials of the real needs of business. This, in turn, contributes to a greater realism in the proposals emanating from the bureaucrats' offices in Brussels.[43]

Some top EEC officials recognize that, as yet, the Community has had little experience in the formulation and implementation of technology strategy. The EEC activities in the area up to now have generally been fairly academic, perhaps somewhat theoretical; probably those mechanisms serving as a link between European industry and the Community process of technology strategy formulation and implementation are not yet sufficiently established. Officials notice a gap between the EEC's interest (to achieve a technological strategy with a European scope and a long-term orientation) and that of European industry, which tends to focus on specific problems and on the short term. They feel that the ESPRIT Program represents new ground in the effort to achieve an improved integration of goals. This could be the result of a learning process. Some Community officials see the ESPRIT model as the seeds of a European parallel to the coordinating function of the Japanese MITI. This learning process might have been easier in the case of the ESPRIT Program, given the aforementioned relatively high concentration of the European electronics industry. Notwithstanding this, some top officials are confident that the coordination model could also be applied in more fragmented sectors, such as that of biotechnology.

The Existence of Effective Leadership

There are few doubts among top Community officials as to the great contribution made by Viscount Etienne Davignon in promoting, developing, and directing the entire process of technology strategy formulation and implementation in Europe.[44] He is also credited with having championed the ESPRIT Program and with having been the inspirer of its implementation model. It should not be forgotten that the ESPRIT Program finances 50% of the cost of projects carried out under its aegis (the other 50% has to be contributed by industry), which means it was necessary to guarantee a prior willingness to cooperate on the part of European industry. The generous budget granted to this program is also probably the result of his power and influence in the EEC, the sums involved comparing favorably with more modest budgets allocated to most Community programs, especially in R&D. Davignon is also credited with the leadership of the "Roundtable of European Industrialists" in whose first meeting he participated in 1983, along with François-Xavier Ortoli, Commissioner with responsibility for Economic Affairs.

It should be pointed out that Viscount Davignon is an expert in European politics and in the internal functioning of the EEC bureaucracy, is knowledgeable about European industry, and enjoys the respect of the bosses of major European firms. It has thus been necessary to have powerful leadership at the apex of the EEC so that steps can be taken in Europe — perhaps for the first time — toward a process of formulation and implementation of "real technology strategy" from the top down. At the same time, a coordination and collaborative model along the lines of the Japanese MITI has been set up. Clearly, the European Coordination model differs from the Japanese model simply because the European economy itself is different: it is a mosaic of countries and political, economic and social systems, as well as being a much more open economy. Davignon, by serving as a catalyst for the start-up of the ESPRIT and Roundtable models, has, without doubt, contributed to the search for an operational model for the implementation of technology strategy in Europe.

Conclusion

A technology strategy model is, indeed, emerging in Europe. It stems from a unanimous perception, that of the danger of being left behind in terms of competition, losing ground to the US and Japan. In order to achieve a sufficient scale, it looks toward a coordination of effort. The mechanisms of formulation and implementation are complex and fragmented. The European model, enshrined in such examples as the ESPRIT Program is similar to what Horwitch[45] describes as Mode III innovation with a large number of linkages of the type described by Horwitch,[46] to which should be added the concept of *supranational-interorganizational linkage* in order to take into account the significant role of the EEC and other supranational institutions. Given the open nature of the European economy, meaning that American and Japanese firms work actively and intensely within it, these linkages go beyond the strict confines of Europe. In this way, although it could be said that European technology strategy is directed largely toward the use of Mode III technological innovation, linkages are also established with Japanese and North American firms.[47] It is even conceivable that European R&D budgets might serve to finance R&D outside Europe in non-European businesses or institutions.[48]

The success of this model will depend on a series of factors, including leadership, the management learning process, and the sharing of results. The leadership aspect, as coming from the EEC, seems to have been a determining factor in transforming a state of mind into properly prepared action. Although Europe is beginning to stir and to build a set of creative and possibly effective approaches to technology strategy, however, it still is unclear how European leadership in the case of technology will evolve in the future, and whether the type of leadership that now exists is best equipped to give further impetus to the process we are studying. It is even possible that such a process can be maintained without explicit leadership.

The second aspect, the management learning process, is also important insofar as there exists no great experience or body of knowledge concerning the application of management to the fluid, fragmented and cooperative process that now characterizes the European situation. Even the most sophisticated strategy formulation and implementation models, which the leading international consulting firms attempt to sell to European business, are more appropriate for directing strategies based on a Mode II technological innovation than for the current situation emerging in Europe. (This is perhaps one of the reasons for the scant success of these models.) The problem is of concern to the academic world in Europe while offering enormous opportunities for research.[49]

The third problem is the sharing of results. Clearly, if this technology strategy process is to meet with any success in Europe, European companies will have to learn to cooperate as well as compete. Community officials and business managers participating in programs such as ESPRIT are concerned by the result-sharing problem, even though it is probable that, at least in the initial stages of cooperation, conflicts will not come to the surface.

In short, Europe is developing its own somewhat unique approach for technology strategy. Indeed, this development represents an important and complex but little-studied phenomenon. It is still too early, however, to predict whether this new technology strategy that is underway can ultimately deal effectively with the severe challenges facing Europe today.

Acknowledgment

The authors would like to express their thanks to the various officials of the European Economic Community for the valuable time they gave in generously cooperating in the writing of this paper, and for making available relevant source material. In particular, the authors acknowledge their debt to Messrs. Richard L. Nobbs of the European Strategic Program for Research and Development in Information Technology (ESPRIT), Albert Saint-Remy of Unite de Concertation pour la Biotechnologie en Europe (CUBE), and Dennis Watson, Head, Task Force for Innovation Coordination.

At the same time, the authors would like to thank those top managers of firms in the Netherlands, Denmark, France, Belgium and Spain, who made time available, especially highlighting the support received from the management of Philips International B.V., Eindhoven, Netherlands.

Notes

1. This situation has been studied repeatedly in academic and business meetings through Europe during the 1980s. For instance: The European Foundation for Management Development organized its annual assembly of 1983 on the topic, "Is Europe Defeated?" (*International Management Development*, Brussels, Autumn, 1983.) The French Employers Confederation and the Paris Chamber of Commerce organized the symposium, "Faisons L'Europe Ensemble," in Paris along the same lines.
2. The Commission of the European Communities, *Eurofutures* (London: Butterworth, 1984), p. 10.
3. Rainald V. Gizycki and Ingrid Schubert, *Microelectronics: A Challenge for Europe's Survival*, a FAST Report (Brussels: Oldenbourg, 1983), p. 25.
4. Rainald V. Gizycki and Ingrid Schubert, *op. cit.*, p. 45.
5. Commission of the European Communities, *Proposal for a Council Decision Adopting the First European Strategic Programme for Research and Development in Information Technologies (ESPRIT)*, COM (83) 258 final (Brussels: Commission of the European Communities, 1983), pp. 7, 8.
6. Edwin Mansfield, *The Economics of Technological Change* (New York: W.W. Norton, 1968), p. 10.
7. Peter Drucker, *Technology, Management and Society* (New York: Harper and Row, 1970), p. 47.
8. Mel Horwitch, "Changing Patterns for Corporate Strategy and Technology Management: The Rise of the Semiconductor and Biotechnology Industries," paper presented at the Mitsubishi Bank Foundation Conference on Business Strategy and Technical Innovations, March 26–29, 1983, Ito City, Japan, p. 1.
9. Wickham C. Skinner, *Manufacturing in the Corporate Strategy* (New York: Wiley, 1978), pp. 81–97.
10. James M. Utterback and William Abernathy, "Patterns of Industrial Innovation," *Technology Review* 80:7 (June–July 1978).
11. Raymond Vernon, ed., *The Technology Factor in International Trade* (New York: National Bureau of Economic Research, 1970); R. Vernon, *Sovereignty at Bay* (New York: Basic Books, 1971); and Duane Kujawa, "Technology Strategy and Industrial Relations: Case Studies of Japanese Multinationals in the United States," *Journal of International Business Studies*, Winter 1983, p. 9.
12. Derek F. Abell, *Defining the Business* (Englewood Cliffs, N.J.: Prentice Hall, 1980), p. 17.
13. Michael E. Porter, "The Technological Dimension of Competitive Strategy," working paper no. 82-19, Graduate School of Business Administration, Harvard University, and Roland L. Roehrich, "The Relationship Between Technological and Business Innovation," *The Journal of Business Strategy* 5:2 (Fall 1984), pp. 60–63.
14. A summarized description of models can be seen in Christer Karlsson, "The Determination of Technology Strategy," *International Management Development*, Spring 1985, p. 16.
15. Mel Horwitch and Kiyonori Sakakibara, "The Changing Strategy: Technology Relationship in Technology-Based Industries: A Comparison of the United States and Japan," paper presented at the Annual Conference of the Strategic Management Society, October 27–29, Paris, France.
16. Hakan Hakasson and Jeus Laage-Hellman, "Developing a Network R&D Strategy," *Journal of Product Innovation Management* (1984), pp. 224–237.
17. Michael A. McGinnis and Robert Ackelsberg, "Effective Innovation Management: Missing Link in Strategic Planning," *The Journal of Business Strategy* 4:1 (Summer 1983), pp. 59–66.
18. T. Burns and G.M. Stalker, *The Management of Innovations* (Tavistock Publications Ltd., 1961).

19. R.L. Daft and S.W. Becker, *Innovation in Organizations* (New York: Elsevier North-Holland, Inc., 1978).

20. L.G. Mohr, "Determinants of Innovation in Organization," *The American Political Science Review* (1969), pp. 111–126.

21. H.A. Shepard, "Innovation Resisting and Innovation Producing Organizations," *The Journal of Business* (1969), pp. 470–477.

22. J.M. Utterback, "The Process of Technological Innovation Within the Firm," *Academy of Management Journal* (1971), pp. 75–88.

23. Harald Hotze, "Reshaping European Industry," *International Management*, January 1985, p. 20; and Pedro Nueno, "Technology Cooperation in Europe," Symposium Faisons L'Europe Ensemble, Paris, Palais des Cougies, October 11–12, 1983.

24. Case: N.V. Philips' Gloeilampenfabrieken, The Tessenderlo Plant, 9-679-082, Harvard Business School, Boston, MA.

25. Personal interviews by the authors in The Netherlands, Denmark, France and Spain.

26. Commission of the European Communities, Directorate General for Science, Research and Development, *The FAST Programme*, Vol. 2 (Brussels: Commission of the European Communities, 1982), p. 22.

27. Several countries inside and outside the EEC (Japan, Canada, US, Sweden, The Netherlands, France, Spain, etc.) have created structures to formulate or influence technology strategy: Japan (1967) created the Agency for Science and Technology attached to the cabinet of the Prime Minister. The US created the Office of Technology Assessment in 1973. The Netherlands (1973) created the Scientific Council for Governmental Policy; Sweden, in 1973, established the Secretariat for Prospective Studies related to the government and Parliament; in 1983 the Spanish Parliament approved the National Electronic and Information Plan, in 1985, the Law of Science, and it is soon expected to approve the National Biotechnology Plan.

28. Several institutions have been created in different countries by national or regional governments to apply venture capital approaches. In Spain, the CDTI (Center for Development of Industrial Technology) is an important government agency that offers loans to companies for R&D projects; these loans must be paid back only if the project succeeds, and on the basis of a royalty on sales of the products obtained as a result of the research.

29. Ira Magaziner and Robert Riech, *Minding America's Business* (New York: Harcourt, 1982).

30. Pedro Nueno, "Industry and Technology Policy in Old Industrialized Regions," paper presented in the meeting on Industrial Policy in Old European Industrialized Regions, Brussels, January 23–24, 1984.

31. Commission of the European Communities, *Vade-Mecum of Contract Research* (Luxembourg: Office Publications of the European Communities, 1984), p. 2.

32. *Ibid.*, p. 1.

33. *Ibid.*, p. 2.

34. Computed by the authors from the list of all R&D programs and actions which were in progress in May 1984. Additional programs or program extensions could be approved and funded within the period 1984–87.

35. Commission of the European Communities, Directorate General for Science, Research and Development, Joint Research Center, FAST, *The FAST Programme*, vol. I (Brussels: Commission of the European Communities, 1982), pp. 191–194.

36. *The FAST Programme*, vol. I, p. 203–208.

37. Commission of the European Communities, *Official Documents on the ESPRIT Programme*, C231, Vol. XXVI (Brussels: Commission of the European Communities, 1984).

38. Commission of the European Communities, "Proposals for a Council Decision" adopting a multiannual research program of the European Economic Community in the field of Biotechnology (1985–89), COM (84), 230 Final (Brussels: Commission of the European Communities, 1984).

39. COST Secretariat, *COST* (Brussels: COST Secretariat, 1981).

40. Harald Hotze, *Reshaping European Industry*, *op. cit.*, p. 23.

41. Roy Eales, "Europe's Industrialists Revive the European Dream," *Multinational INFO*, Institute for Research and Information on Multinationals, no. 7 (February 1985), p. 4.

42. In the field of biotechnology, for instance, see Commission of the European Communities, "Biotechnology: The Community's Role" (background note: national initiatives for the support of biotechnology), COM (83) 328 Final/2 (Brussels: Commission of the European Communities, 1983); and Commission of the European Communities, Directorate General for Science, Research and Development, "A Community Strategy for Biotechnology in Europe," FAST occasional papers, no. 62 (Brussels: FAST, 1983).

43. A specialized lobby firm interviewed by the authors explained that the processes of the different EEC bodies involved in the formulation and implementation of technology strategy are so complex that even large companies utilize the services of specialized firms well connected to the key EEC bureaucracy. These firms guide company executives and scientists in the preparation and negotiation of proposals.

44. Viscount Etienne Davignon ended his term as Industrial Commissioner of the European Economic Community in December 1984.

45. Mel Horwitch, "The Changing Strategy-Technology Relationship in Technology-Based Industries: A Com-

parison of the United States and Japan," *op. cit.*, p. 2.

46. *Ibid.*, p. 6.

47. Harald Hotze, *op. cit.*, for a list of technological "links" between European companies and US and Japanese counterparts.

48. These are some forms of R&D for which this possibility already exists in the EEC and in the member and non-member states.

49. The Meeting of Deans and Directors of European Management Schools of January 9–11, 1985, focused on this problem. (Implications of New Technological Developments for Management and Management Education). The conclusions of the meeting stressed the importance of researching aspects such as intercompany deals on technology and top management technology strategy. (*Proceedings* of the Conference published by EFMD, Rue Washington, 40, B-1050, Brussels.)

Innovation and Corporate Strategy

Managed Chaos

James Brian Quinn

ABSTRACT. *Because major technological changes tend to progress in a highly probabilistic, tumultuous, interactive fashion — driven by a few champions — corporate innovation programs must be designed and managed accordingly. Based on a 2½-year study of large, innovative enterprises, this article suggests how some of the world's most innovative companies interlink careful strategic planning concepts with some novel organizational and motivational approaches to achieve their purposes. Neither structured formality nor unstructured chaos works well alone. Innovative companies seem to evolve a sophisticated approach to "managed chaos," which recognizes the realities of how major technological innovations evolve, and harnesses this process to corporate needs. While some general principles apply, the particular strengths, style, goals and competitive situation of each company may dictate very different specific solutions. But experience suggests certain common threads whose adoption increases the probability of succeeding.*

The competitive environment facing large US and European corporations has probably changed more in the past 25 years than in the preceding 100. In earlier years, most such corporations operated either in imperialistic situations or in islands of competition involving primarily their own domestic markets, a few large domestic competitors with similar cost structures, generally supportive governments, technologies which could be developed in depth and protected for substantial periods, and/or special access to low-cost capital which allowed overwhelming scale economies or barriers to market entry. Now virtually all their markets and competitors are international in scale; domestic governments are often adversaries (on capital, tax, environmental or welfare issues); foreign governments are direct competitors; technologies and capital move rapidly across world borders[1]; and individual countries' materials costs, labor costs, monetary exchange rates, or intervention strategies create a bizarre array of cost patterns not present in the domestic market place.

How can a modern corporation produce domestically in a world where its capital costs are twice those of some competitors (Japan), its labor costs are 10 to 20 times higher than others (the LDCs),[2] its nation's safety and environmental standards are

James Brian Quinn is a well-known scholar, author and consultant on strategic planning, entrepreneurship and innovation. He is Buchanan Professor of Management at Amos Tuck Graduate School of Business, Dartmouth College, and has participated on numerous teams, nationally and internationally, for the National Academies of Science and Engineering.

among the world's highest, and its raw materials and energy bases have moved overseas. Strategically there are only a few options:

- Anticipating and servicing specific customers' needs better than anyone else in the world;
- Innovating faster and more continuously than all competitors; and
- Leveraging one's own capabilities by accessing and utilizing the world's best external science, technology and information sources.

To do this requires that companies integrate their research, technology, production, marketing and innovation management practices in a way few have achieved. Several streams of research suggest certain critical dimensions.

A Planning Perspective

Management research has defined well the formal methodologies for effectively aligning research and development activities with corporate goals.[3] The most successful enterprises seem to:

- Establish broad but challenging overall company objectives in light of predicted long-term economic, sociological and technological developments;
- Determine what specific unique strategy the overall company and each of its major divisions will use in effecting these objectives;
- Rank and balance research programs and projects into patterns which match these needs and deal with anticipated threats and opportunities in the external environment; and
- Develop clear mechanisms and a supporting motivational environment to transfer results from research to operations.

Continuous *minor changes in existing technologies* are often an important component in a technical strategy. These can and generally should be accomplished within such relatively planned frameworks. But such planning does not provide sufficient links for technology and strategy in today's complex world.

A Historical Perspective

Historians of technology have thoroughly documented that most *major technological advances* occur not in the linear mode suggested above, but in a relatively chaotic sequence of events typically involving an early vision; numerous fits, starts and lapses in progress; random interactions with the outside world; frequent intuitive insights and personal risk-taking; and even some lucky breaks which ultimately lead to success.[5] While in retrospect a technology may seem to progress (worldwide) doggedly up a Gaussian curve toward its ultimate theoretical limits,[6] more detailed observers see a series of "relatively small steps marked by an occasional obstacle and by constant random breakthroughs interacting across laboratories and borders."[7]

The unraveling of DNA's structure first followed a convoluted and somewhat disjointed route through various nations' biology, organic chemistry, x-ray crystallography and mathematics laboratories until its rather rapid, Nobel prize-winning conception as a spiral staircase of matched base pairs.[8] Then years of painstaking and highly individualistic research on gene structures and enzymes went through alternating periods of optimism and discouragement before the possibility of practical recombinant DNA suddenly emerged from Boyer and Cohen's 1972 discussions over sandwiches after a Hawaiian meeting. And now — almost 3 decades after Watson and Crick's insights and 12 years after Boyer and Cohen's first experiments — rDNA's first commercial applications are still moving forward in fits of insight and frustration as its expected major uses (like self-fertilizing plants, interferon, or commercial waste decomposition) constantly encounter new problems and create new surprises in their struggle toward the marketplace.

Companies seeking strategic advantage through significant technological innovation need to recognize the tumultuous, long-term realities of how this process operates, and design specific organizations and management practices to motivate and guide it. This paper is based on a two-and-one-half-year study of how some of the world's most innovative large companies stimulate such activities, yet maintain the practical controls so essential to efficient current operations.

Time Horizons — Vision

Perhaps the most difficult issue for most enterprises to overcome is the time horizon needed for major innovations.[9] Most radical innovations — *e.g.*, jet aircraft engines, float glass, recombinant DNA, hovercraft, xerography, nuclear power, etc. — take over a decade from first discovery to net positive cash flows.[10] In my sample, delays ranged from three to 25 years.

For example, in the late 1930's Russell Marker was working on steroids called sapogenins, which make a soap-like foam in water. In the process he found a technique that would degrade one of these, diosgenin, into the female sex hormone progesterone. Marker found that diosgenin was abundant in certain Mexican yams. By processing about ten tons of these in rented and borrowed lab space, he extracted some 4 pounds of diosgenin, and in 1944 started a tiny company, Syntex, producing steroids for the laboratory market. But it was not until 1957 that Searle started marketing a derivative, norethynodril, as a menstrual regulator — with a specific warning against "possible contraceptive activity." In 1962, over 23 years after Marker's early research, Syntex obtained FDA approval for its oral contraceptive.

Even smaller extensions of technology typically take two to five years from initiation to first positive rewards. Such delays are often anathema — to public companies, who gauge their success against quarterly reports of profitability, to managers who are rotated in two-year patterns, and to public laboratories dependent upon annual or biennial elections for their support.[11] Yet short time horizons need not be the norm. All the innovative enterprises in my sample had found ways to deal with this problem.

Long time horizons can occur in organizations for a variety of reasons. In some, the very nature of the product creates such views. Aircraft manufacturers, pharmaceutical companies, public utilities, electrical generation equipment producers, forest products companies, shipbuilders, etc., all have very long operating time horizons. Successful companies in these fields must develop internal management systems to plan and control on multiple-year horizons, or they fail. Their corporate cultures and financial sources accept such horizons as given. But such companies are not all innovative. Long time horizons alone do not lead to innovativeness.

Vision

Continuous innovation occurs largely because a few key executives have a broad vision of what their organizations can accomplish for the world and lead their enterprises toward it. They appreciate the role of innovation in achieving their goals and consciously manage their concerns' value systems and atmospheres to support it. Because familiarity fosters understanding and decreases one's fear of risk in a situation, technical people (or those who have personally participated in successful innovations) are often those who create such supportive atmospheres. But — as the nontechnical top managers of Genentech, IBM, Pilkington, Elf Aquitaine, AT&T, Merck and others in my sample amply illustrate — executive vision is more important than one's functional background.

Innovative managements — whether technical or not — project clear long-term visions for their organizations that go beyond simple economic performance measurements.[12] For example:

> Intel's chairman, Gordon Moore, says: "We intend [for Intel] to be the outstandingly successful company in our industry. We intend to be a leader in this revolutionary [semi-conductor] technology that is changing the way the world is run." Young people attracted by Intel's goals and style responded, "It's great to say you work at Intel. You know you're with the best. . . . There's a real pride in being first, in being on the frontier. You know you are part of something very big — very important."
>
> Genentech's original plan states: "We expect to be the first company to commercialize the [rDNA] technology, and we plan to build a major profitable corporation by manufacturing and marketing needed products that benefit mankind. . . . The future uses of genetic engineering are far reaching and many. Micro-organisms could be engineered to produce proteins to meet the world's food needs or to produce antibodies to fight viral infections. Any product produced by a living organism is eventually within the company's reach."[13]

Such visions, vigorously supported, have many practical applications. They attract quality people to the company, and give focus to their creative and entrepreneurial drives. People who share common values and goals can work independently, self-coordinating their activities without detailed controls. And they are more motivated to achieve goals they generally believe in. Overarching goals and values help power growth by concentrating on the actions which lead to profitability, rather than on profitability itself. Such visions establish a realistic time-frame for innovation and, properly presented externally, attract the kind of investors who will support it. In essence, they provide the rationale for that ultimate expression of stockholder confidence and patience, high P/E ratios.

Market-Goal Orientation

Innovative companies then consciously anchor their visions to the practical realities of the marketplace. Each company develops specific techniques adapted to its particular style and strategy, but two elements are always present: (1) a strong market orientation at the very top of the company, and (2) explicit mechanisms to force market-technical interactions at lower levels. For example:

> Sony's Chairman Morita, who has personally started several of its most innovative ventures, purposely seeks informal settings where he can meet with and understand the lifestyles of trend-setting younger people. Soon after technical people are hired, Sony cycles them through weeks of retail selling. Sony engineers become sensitive to the ways retail sales practices, displays, and non-quantifiable customer preferences affect success.[14]

> Bell Laboratories has an Operating Company Assignment Program (OCAP) to rotate its researchers through AT&T-Western development and producing facilities. And until the AT&T break-up, Bell Laboratories maintained a rigorous Engineering Complaint System through which it collected technical problems and inquiries from its operating companies. These inquiries *had* to receive an "action response" within a month, *i.e.*, Bell Labs *had* to specify how it could solve or would attempt to resolve the problem and notify the operating company (in writing) of its action.

From top management to bench levels in my sample's "most innovative" companies, executives' primary focus seemed to be on opportunistically seeking and solving customers' emerging problems. For example, rather than follow many others companies' practices by cutting back or shutting down operations in the 1981–82 recession, Intel started its "20% solution." Key members of the professional staff agreed to work an extra day a week for several months to bring out new products earlier and to solve customer problems in ways that maintained Intel's own employment. Other examples follow.

A Unique Strategic Focus

How each enterprise can best satisfy identified needs depends on its own particular strengths and style—and the characteristics of the field it is in. Successful innovation managements carefully conceptualize the role they want innovation to play in their strategies, and organize for that purpose. This has led to quite different alignments in various companies based on their particular technologies, skills, resources, and desired risk patterns. Several distinctive strategies will make the point:

Extensions of Customers' R&D. Some suppliers of technical specialities to original equipment manufacturers (OEMs) regard their own technologists as extensions of their customers' R&D programs. Typically the supplier has knowledge depth in areas different from its customers — *i.e.*, a chemical specialties producer like Dewey & Almy or a semi-conductor specialist like Intel supplying a mechanical OEM. Such suppliers develop strong technical networks to discover and understand customer needs in depth and try to have their solutions designed into the customers' products. These companies maintain flexible applied technology groups working close to the marketplace — and even on customer premises. All technology is kept highly proprietary. They have quickly expandable production facilities and a cutting edge technology (not necessarily basic research) group that allows rapid selection of the best available technologies to solve problems.

Basic Research Enterprises. Some companies like Genentech, Merck, or Hoffman LaRoche have been built on basic research strategies. These companies offer researchers better equipped laboratories, higher pay, and often more freedom than universities in order to attract top flight people. To make sure their people are on the cutting edge of science, they allow researchers to publish extensively (after appropriate patent applications, if relevant), participate in meetings, and develop wide colleague networks externally. They further leverage their internal spending through research grants, clinical grants, and direct research relationships with outside groups throughout the world. These companies want a clear understanding of possible alternatives and a preemptive position in the sciences underlying the product before they invest $20 to $50 million to clear and produce a new drug. But their basic science activities must also be coupled with elaborate precautions to ensure that the drug is safe and effective in use and controllable in manufacture. Hence their structures are designed to place them at the frontiers of science, but to be quite conservative in animal testing, clinical evaluations and production control.

Entrepreneurial Start Ups. Some companies, like Hewlett Packard and 3M, have strategies to develop product lines from a series of small, discrete, free-standing new product concepts. These companies form units akin to entrepreneurial start ups. Each tends to be a small team, led by a product champion, in relatively low cost "incubator" facilities, where overheads are kept to a minimum. These companies allow many different proposals to come forward and test them — experimentally and interactively — as early as possible in the marketplace. Their control systems try to spot and prevent significant early losses on any entry. Like venture capitalists they look for their high gains on a few successful products. But, unlike venture capitalists, they also try to blend their less successful, smaller, individual entries into product lines their existing channels or facilities can support.

Major Systems Innovations. Other companies (like AT&T, the aircraft companies, or the oil majors) have to innovate large scale systems that only pay back if they last for decades. These concerns make very long term needs and competitive forecasts, with all possible precision. They often start several alternate designs in parallel to be as sure as possible of selecting the right technologies at the last moment before commercialization. They extensively test new system and subsystem technologies in actual use before making full-scale commitments. And they frequently sacrifice speed of entry for long-term low cost and reliability.

Many other examples, of course, exist. And even within a single company, individual divisions may have different strategic needs—hence different structures and practices.[15] No single approach to innovation suits all situations.

Managing Chaos

If such formalities were all that is required for innovation, many more companies would be successful at it. The central problem is that innovation—first reduction of an idea to practice—is a process that rarely can be planned and controlled with the kind of analytical certainty managers associate with other operations. Instead, technology tends to advance in a bubbling, intuitive, tumultuous process—more akin to a fermentation vat than a production line.[16] Initial discoveries tend to be highly individualistic and serendipitous, advances chaotic and interactive, and specific outcomes unpredictable and chancy until the very last moment. How can one manage such a process in a large organization?

Multiple Approaches

All innovation is probabilistic. At first, one cannot know whether the desired result can be achieved or which of several possible approaches may dominate the field as it develops. Initial insights can come from almost anywhere—and the right insight can create a whole new industry or offer dominance to its discoverer for years.

> Henry Perkin, trying to synthesize quinine from coal tar, discovered the synthetic purple dye that began the modern chemical industry. Leo Baekeland was looking for a synthetic shellac when he found Bakelite and started the modern plastics industry. A gust of wind, blowing mold on Fleming's cultures, created the antibiotic age. The microcomputer was born because Ted Hoff happened to work on a complex calculator for a Japanese client just when DEC's PDP8 architecture was fresh in his mind. Carl Djerassi's group at Syntex was not looking for an oral contraceptive when it created 19-norprogesterone, the precursor to norethindrome which became the active ingredient in half of all contraceptive pills. Sir Alastair Pilkington was washing dishes when he got the critical insight that led to float glass. And so on.

To increase the probability of some program's succeeding and to multiply the kinds of interactions that lead to success, innovative companies (where possible) encourage several programs to proceed in parallel. Lucky "accidents" are involved in almost all major technological advances. When theory can predict everything, one is in production stages—not development. In fact, Murphy's Law works because engineers design for what they can foresee; hence what fails is what theory did not predict. And it is rare that the interactions of components and subsystems can be predicted over the complete performance envelope of a complex device's anticipated operations. For example, despite thorough theoretical design work, the first high-performance US jet engine literally tore itself to pieces on its test stand.[17] Later, well tested jet engines failed in an Iranian sand storm during the US attempt to rescue its Embassy's personnel held as hostages.

Recognizing these characteristics of development, all of the "most innovative" companies in my sample consciously started several prototype programs in parallel, thinning down the number of alternatives only as probabilities of success approached certainty or costs became prohibitive. Sony, for example, in its video-tape recorder (VTR) program pursued ten different major options, each with two to three subsystem alternatives. Such redundancy helps both in coping with some of the inherent randomness and unpredictability in development and in motivating people through constructive competition. The latter may easily be as important as the former.

Development Shoot-Outs

To gain maximum motivational and information benefits many of these companies consciously structure "shoot-outs" between competing approaches only after they reach advanced prototype stages. Managers find this practice: (1) provides the most objective possible data for decision purposes; (2) decreases risks by making choices as close as possible to the marketplace; and (3) ensures that whatever option wins will move ahead with a committed team behind it. Although anathema to many who worry about presumed *efficiencies* in R&D, greater *effectiveness* in choosing a right solution can easily outweigh "duplication costs." This is likely to be the case when the market genuinely rewards higher performance or when large volumes justify increased technical or cost sophistication. Under these conditions competing approaches can both improve probabilities of success and decrease development times, making parallel development less costly in both the short and long run.

Properly rewarding and reintegrating losing teams is perhaps the most difficult and essential skill in managing competing projects. If the total company is expanding rapidly or if the successful project creates a substantial growth opportunity, competing team members can generally find another interesting program or sign on with the "winner" as it moves toward the marketplace. For the shoot-out system to work continuously, however, executives must create a climate that honors high performance, whether it wins or loses; reabsorbs people quickly into their technical specialities or onto other projects; and accepts and expects rotation among tasks and groups.

At Polaroid during its prolonged growth period it was an honor to work on one of Dr. Land's projects. Many of these grew into the major new product lines of the company with attendant management opportunities. Some specialized technical solutions (like high-performance batteries) became entire new divisions. Many engineers followed products into production, operating production prototype machines at first, then phasing back into development activities or forward into manufacturing management. The R&D organization was described as a "coat rack of talent to be assembled and reassembled on projects as it was needed, but with a base of attractive problems to attack whenever people were not involved on specific task forces." Those who were successful on these projects became the next generation of management at Polaroid.[18]

Small, Flexible Teams

To further enhance motivation, interactiveness, and rapid progress, innovative companies also emphasize small teams working in a relatively independent environment. The optimum number of key players sought per team varies from five to seven. This number seems to provide a critical mass of skills, foster maximum communications,[19] and allow sufficient latitude for individual creativeness and commitment. The epitome of this style is the "skunkworks"—named after "Kelly" Johnson's successful group at Lockheed—in which small teams of engineers, technicians and designers are placed together with no intervening organizational barriers to developing a new product or process from concept to commercial prototype stages.

Innovative European groups (like Pilkington Brothers or Elf Aquitaine) or Japanese companies (like Sony or Honda) also used this approach. Interestingly, Japan's much publicized *Ringii* decision-making was not evident in these latter situations. Sony's founder, Mr. Ibuka, or his technical successor, Mr. Kihara, participated directly with their design groups, and made rapid "on the spot" decisions at key junctures. Soichiro Honda was known for working with his engineering and design groups and emphasizing his own views by shouting at his engineers and occasionally even popping them with a wrench.[20]

Progress in technology is largely determined by the number of successful experiments made per unit time. Skunkworks help eliminate bureaucratic delays, allow fast unfettered communication, and permit the quick turnarounds and decisions that stimulate rapid advance. To further enhance fast, effective decision-making, many of the most innovative enterprises observed also tried to structure flat organizations to decrease the number of organizational layers between the bench worker and the top. By keeping total division sizes below 400, close communications can be maintained with only two intervening decision layers to the top. In units much larger than this, people quickly lose touch with the total concept of their product or process, bureaucracies grow, and projects must go through more and more formal screens to survive. Since it takes a chain of "yesses" to approve a project as it moves to the top and only one "no" to kill it, jeopardy multiplies as management layers increase.

Interactive Learning Processes

But the most innovative enterprises go even further in structuring interactiveness. They consciously tap into multiple outside sources of technological capability. The first of these is their own customers. Many studies have shown that demand and technology often drive one another. Von Hipple[21] suggests that over 50% of all innovation in some industries (like electronics) is performed by customers. In others (like textiles) materials or equipment suppliers provide most of the innovation. In still others (like biotechnology) universities are dominant, while foreign sources strongly contribute to industries such as pharmaceuticals, foods, or environmental controls.

No company or research group can spend more than a small portion of the world's (approximately $200 billion) R&D budget. Yet scientific knowledge and technological advances from outside sources and seemingly unrelated fields—like biology and medicine's increasing intersections with electronics—often interact to create totally new concepts or opportunities important to an enterprise. Recognizing this, many concerns have active strategies to develop information for trading with outside research or technology groups, and special teams to cultivate these sources.[22] Large Japanese companies, of course, have been notably effective at this. So have such diverse US companies as DuPont, AT&T, Apple Computer, Johnson & Johnson, and Genentech. Wholly new relationships in which large companies participate—as joint venturers, consortium members, limited partners, guarantors of first markets, venture capitalists, or spin-off equity holders—have begun to rival the imagination and variety of structures used in entrepreneurial start ups. These represent some of the most exciting new dimensions for corporate strategies in the current decade.

Champions, Experts and Rewards

Many studies have emphasized the essential role of a "determined champion" in overcoming the many soul-wrenching disappointments and setbacks major innovation always seems to encounter.[23] In large organizations, in particular, the process seems long term, ambiguous, uncertain, frustrating, and debilitating beyond belief. It seems to be in the nature of both the receiving organizations (production units, customers, or one's own peers) to actively adapt to resist change. Often only a fanatic can survive the strain. And even some of them ultimately give up.

> These frustrations were so intense that Armstrong (creator of FM), Carothers (synthetic fibers), and Diesel (the diesel engine) committed suicide before their great inventions reached full commercial success. Goddard (champion of rocketry), Whittle (jet aircraft engines), Carlson (Xerox), Sikorski (helicopters), Ibuka (video tape recorders), and Ovshinski (amorphous semi-conductors) are typical of those who pour frustrating decades into their radical innovations before they become profitable.

Fortunately their fanaticism makes innovator-entrepreneurs underestimate the length of time and obstacles to success. Time horizons for radical innovations (averaging at least 12 years) make them essentially irrational from a calculated financial investment (present value) viewpoint. For these reasons individual champions (or fanatics) are the heart and soul of most small start-up entrepreneurial ventures, substituting sweat capital (or entrepreneurial rent) for actual dollar investments.

Similarly, a few such people almost always drive any innovation in a larger enterprise — in all cases in my study. But rarely can a single individual carry out an entire innovation alone. A champion desperately needs other expertise and support — both business and technical — at crucial times. Some of the most difficult problems for large organizations are: (1) how to tolerate and nurture the kinds of off-beat, driven personalities who tend to become champions; and (2) how to reward both champions and experts appropriately.

Professional Venture Teams?

Because so many large enterprises fail on both counts, cities like Boston, Minneapolis and San Francisco are surrounded by successful companies started by erstwhile champions not handled properly by their former employers. Recognizing the joint skills and motivation problems involved, many companies try to assign identified innovations to "new venture teams" with the professional (engineering, marketing and finance) skills to see them through. But these teams rarely succeed if the actual champion is not a member (preferably the head) of the team. Texas Instruments made a study of some 40 of its own innovations, and found no projects which were successful where management had chosen the team head. Innovations seem to be much like human babies. For a high probability of success an innovation needs a mother (champion) who loves it emotionally and will stay with it when others would give up, a father (authority figure with resources) who can support it, and pediatricians (experts) who can see it through technical difficulties. Unfortunately many companies assign the task only to their pediatricians.

Rewards pose a special complexity. Most large concerns do not feel they can offer internal innovators the millions of dollars they might make if they successfully build their own companies. Lack of personal investment by the innovator and concerns about "fair play to others" are the reasons most often cited. Yet the few concerns that have made innovative leaders very rich do not seem to have suffered inordinately. And, of course, those who do nothing are protected by the fact that losses caused by potential innovators leaving (or not performing) do not appear on income statements.

The most innovative companies do recognize that innovative champions tend to work for more than just monetary rewards.[24] They try to offer innovators significant personal recognition, independence in research, appropriate power or visibility within the company or in the division exploiting the innovation, or that most cherished of technical incentives — the right to a major role in the next big innovation.[25] Some examples will suggest the kinds of specific rewards offered:

> Sony gives "a small but significant" percentage of a new product's sales to its innovating teams. Pilkington, IBM and 3M's top executives have often been chosen from those who earlier headed successful new product entries. Intel let its Magnetic Memory Group operate like a small company with special performance rewards and simulated stock options. GE, Syntex and UTC have actively helped internal champions of "non-related" product innovations establish new companies and have taken equity positions in their enterprises. And so on.

Increasingly, however, companies are supplementing such recognition with much larger financial awards to keep their most productive people from jumping outside.

Planning Versus Chaos

While understanding and permitting the essential chaos of innovation, effective managers also channel its main directions. As has been suggested, formal planning has severe limitations in this area, particularly in the early stages of the process. For example, formal market analyses may be very useful for product line extensions, but they are often quite misleading when applied to radical innovations.[26]

Such studies said: "Haloid would never sell more than 5000 xerographic machines"; Intel's microprocessor "would never sell more than 10% as many units as there were minicomputers"; Sony's transistor radios and miniature television sets "would fail in the marketplace." All were big winners. Yet more heralded concepts (like Hovercrafts, bio-engineered insulin, and Josephson-effect devices) have yet to fulfill their projections. Many of industry's largest failures were actually over-planned and -researched on paper (like Ford's Edsel, IBM's FS system, and FAA's SST) rather than interactively developed with genuine customer feedback.

Frequently, neither innovators, market researchers nor users can quite visualize a totally new product's real potential. Initial markets often depend on opportunistic adaptations to specific unsuspected needs.

Edison's lights first appeared on ships and in baseball parks. Astro Turf was intended to convert the flat roofs and asphalt playgrounds of city schools into more humane environments. Recording English language programs for Japanese schools was the unexpected first market for audio tape recorders. The hovercraft only became profitable when its original "amphibian" use concept was abandoned and rigid "side skirts" were extended into the water. Graphite and boron fibers unexpectedly found their major uses in sporting equipment. And so on.

Recognizing the limits of early-stage marketing forecasts, more innovative companies tend to move to interactive testing in lead customers' hands as soon as possible. They both benefit from some of these customers' own innovative ideas and learn what the product's actual use and desirability characteristics will be.

Hewlett Packard, 3M, Sony, and Raychem — among the most sophisticated diversifying innovators encountered — specifically acknowledge the complexity of assessing new markets and the benefits of highly interactive relationships with customers during development. They frequently introduce radical new products through small teams closely participating with lead customers, learning from them, and rapidly modifying designs and entry strategies around this information.

Chaos Within Milestones

Instead of relying on detailed plans and control systems, innovative top managements—like venture capitalists—tend to administer primarily by helping establish goals, selecting key people, and defining certain critical limits or decision points at which they will intervene. As technology leads or market needs emerge, they set a few—most crucial—performance targets or concept limits.

Pilkington's Board stipulated that "the float glass process must obsolete all existing plate processes in order to go ahead." Data General's management announced "no mode bit" for the Eagle computer. Mr. Ibuka, Sony's chairman, first set a target of "comparable performance with Ampex but at ¼ the cost" for Sony's first videotape recorder; then shortly thereafter targeted an "industrial video cassette recorder for ¹⁄₁₀ the price"; and finally envisioned the "first *home* video recorder at ⅓ the industrial cassette's price." Each of these was a clear target, but an incredible challenge at the time.

These managements then allow their technical units to decide how to achieve these, subject to defined constraints and program reviews at crucial junctures. Early bench-scale projects may at first pursue many options with little attempt to integrate them all into a total program. Only after key variables are understood—and perhaps measured and demonstrated in lab models—may more precise planning be meaningful. Even then many factors may remain unknown, and competition can continue to thrive in pursuit of solutions. At agreed-on review points, however, only those options that can clear defined performance hurdles or milestones may continue (see Figure 1). But managers may still continue a few other options as

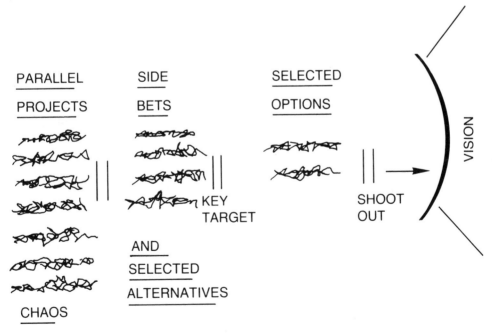

FIGURE 1. Somewhat Orderly Tumult

small-scale "side bets" in case something goes wrong. In a surprising number of cases, these alternatives prove successful when the planned options fail.

As the program approaches ultimate exploitation, uncertainty decreases, and costs escalate. This is where formal planning, using the full array of program planning, economic evaluation, and progress monitoring techniques can pay high dividends. By then, however, incremental approaches[27] have built the information bases, options, certainty of outcomes, motivation, comfort levels in management, and political power bases necessary for the program to compete and succeed against options more familiar—and hence seemingly less risky—to the enterprise.

Complex Portfolio Planning

Such approaches increase the possibility of individual innovative programs developing successfully. But in the turmoil of a number of such endeavors proceeding throughout the organization, top managers also need some way to balance the requirements and benefits of current lines against those of intermediate-horizon and future prospects. While it is inappropriate to detail such a planning system here, this calls for a complex dual matrix planning approach (highlighted in Figure 2) in which the total corporate strategy is broken down into its key thrusts. To the extent possible, these are assigned to individual divisions (the vertical vectors in Figure 2), with differential investment returns defined for each division to allow them the time horizons to fulfill their roles. For example, divisions charged with developing the company's ten-year future markets cannot be expected to make the same returns (on a present value basis) as divisions charged with exploiting existing technologies. And so on.

But there will also be thrusts that cut across divisions (the horizontal vectors in Figure 2). These require that each appropriate division devote *enough* resources to fulfill its share of that thrust. If each division merely ranks and supports programs in terms of returns to that division, it will tend to eliminate or underfund needed corporate strategic programs, particularly longer-run or risky activities. It is essential that strategy override short term (tactical) or divisional (local) priorities. Corporate strategic controls must see that *enough* resources are devoted to each major thrust, even if this means divisions must perform some projects with lower seeming (divisional) returns than some projects which must be rejected. All this requires a much more complex concept of portfolio planning than the often discussed and popular Boston Consulting Group "four box" matrix. Figure 2 is a simplified version of the practices many large innovative companies use for this purpose.

Conclusion

In successfully managing innovation, such formal techniques are important to help provide balance, adequate time horizons, and reasonable overall resource allocations to protect both the enterprise's present and future needs. They are essential to good strategy, but not sufficient for the purpose.

Because major technical changes tend to progress in a highly probabilistic, tumultuous, interactive fashion—driven by a few champions—innovation programs

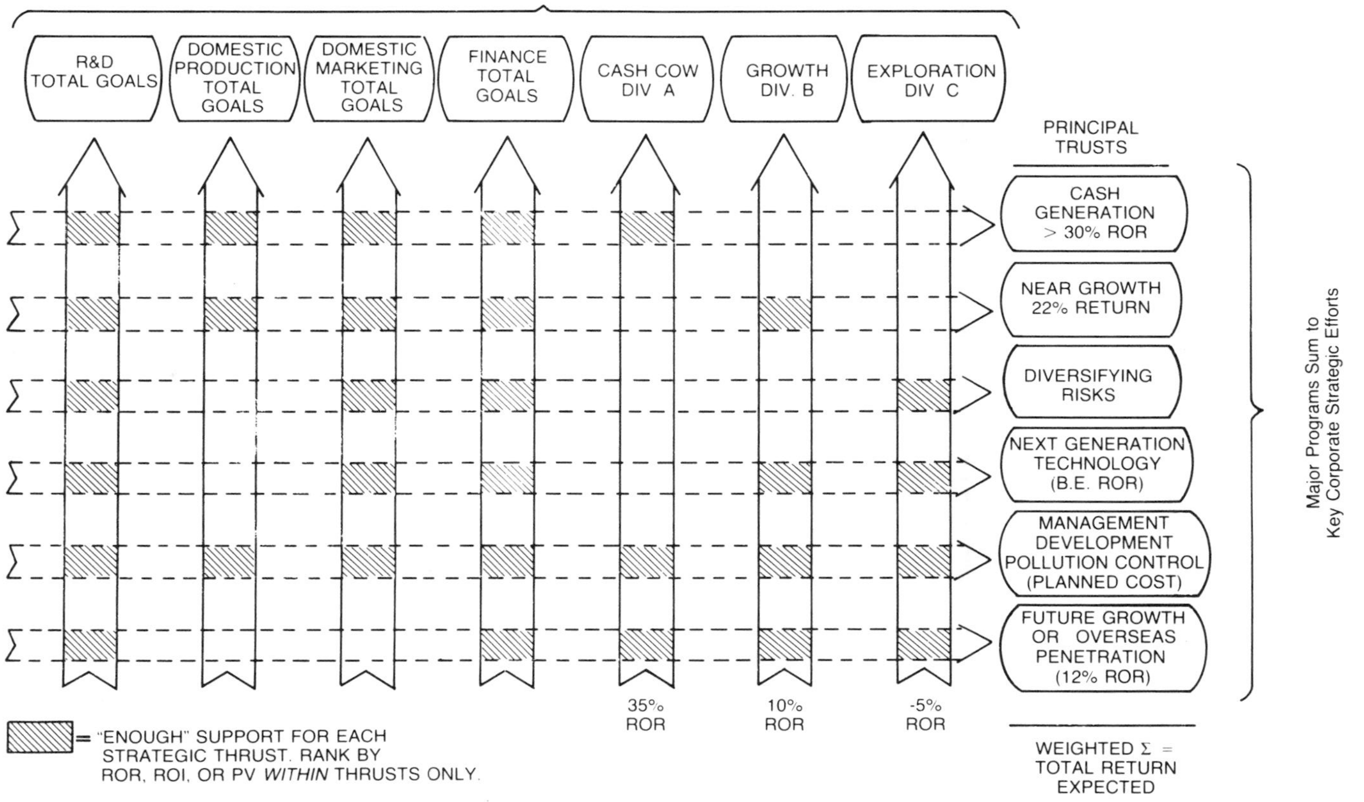

FIGURE 2. Division Goals Sum to Corporate Strategic Goals

The total strategy is divided into 6-10 Principal Strategic Thrusts. Each of these has a different minimum hurdle rate (or allowed cost total) for its programs. Each division's or function's plans and budgets must show *sufficient* support for its share of that strategic thrust. When an entire thrust cannot be assigned to a specific division, efforts are coordinated across divisions to obtain the desired total corporate impact. Each division has its own expected rate of return within which some programs can achieve higher and others lower returns. The weighted sum of all programs' and divisions' returns must meet the overall corporation's targets.

must be designed accordingly. This article suggests how some of the world's most innovative companies interlink careful strategic planning concepts with some novel organizational and motivational approaches to achieve these dual purposes. Neither structured formality nor unstructured chaos will work well alone. Innovative companies seem to evolve a sophisticated approach to "managed chaos" which recognizes the realities of how major technological innovations evolve and harnesses this process to corporate needs. While some general principles apply, the particular strengths, style, goals and competitive situation of each company may dictate very different specific solutions. But experience suggests certain common threads whose adoption increases the probability of succeeding.

Notes

1. R. Vernon and W. Davidson, *Foreign Production of Technology Intensive Products* (Washington, DC: National Science Foundation, 1979).
2. For specific data, see: J.B. Quinn, "Overview of the Current Status of US Manufacturing: Optimizing US Manufacturing" in *U.S. Leadership in Manufacturing* (Washington, DC: National Academy of Engineering, 1983).
3. M. Tushman and W. Moore, *Readings in the Management of Innovation* (Boston: Pitman Publishing, 1982) perhaps offers the best current single collection of these sources.
4. See J.B. Quinn, "Long Range Planning of Industrial Research," *Harvard Business Review*, July–August 1961, and "Transferring Research Results to Operations," *Harvard Business Review*, January–February 1964, for a more complete delineation of key issues and approaches.
5. D. DeSola Price, "Of Sealing Wax and String," *Natural History*, January 1984, offers an eminent technological historian's view of this process. J. Jewkes, D. Sawyers and R. Stillerman, *The Sources of Invention* (London: MacMillan & Co., 1958) is perhaps the first classical presentation of this theme.
6. J. Fisher and R. Pry, "A Simple Substitution Model of Technological Change," monograph. 1981. J. Birnbaum, "Computers: A Survey of Trends and Limitations," *Science* February 12, 1982. R. Ayres, "Envelope Curve Forecasting" in J. Bright, ed., *Technological Forecasting for Industry and Government* (New York: Prentice Hall, 1968).
7. T. Hughes, "The Inventive Continuum," *Science '84*, p. 83.
8. J. Watson, *The Double Helix* (New York: Athenaeum Publishing Co., 1968) offers an excellent narrative of many crucial events in this sequence.
9. R.C. Dean, "The Temporal Mismatch—Innovation's Pace vs. Management's Time Horizon," *Research Management*, May 1974.
10. Battelle Memorial Laboratories, "Science, Technology, and Innovation," Report to the National Science Foundation, Columbus, Ohio, 1973.
11. See R. Hayes and D. Garvin, "Managing As If Tomorrow Really Mattered," *Harvard Business Review*, May–June 1982; and S. Ramo, *America's Technology Slip* (New York: John Wiley & Sons, 1980).
12. T. Kono, *Strategy and Structure of Japanese Enterprises* (Armonk, NY: M. Sharpe, Inc., 1984).
13. From case studies: *Intel Corporation and Genentech Inc.*, copyright, J.B. Quinn, Amos Tuck School, Dartmouth College, 1981.
14. N. Lyons, *The Sony Vision* (New York: Crown Publishers, 1976).
15. A. Chandler, *Strategy and Structure: Chapters in the History of American Industrial Enterprise* (Cambridge, MA: MIT Press, 1962) provides the classic study suggesting that for effectiveness, structure must follow strategy.
16. D. Schon, *Technology and Change* (New York: Delacorte Press, 1967) was among the first to view the management implications of this reality.
17. In *Herman the German* (New York: W.C. Morrow Publishing, 1984), Gerhard Neumann, the longtime head of GE's aircraft engine division, describes this event and other aspects of managing development in his company.
18. M. Olshaker, *The Instant Image* (New York: Stein & Day, 1978).
19. My colleague, Victor McGee, has calculated the total number of one-way channels of communications in a group as $n[2^{(n-1)} - 1]$, which shows a large increase in channels from 75 to 1016 as numbers move from five to eight persons in a group.

20. T. Sakiya, *Honda Motors: The Men, The Management, The Machines* (Tokyo: Kodansha International Ltd., 1982).
21. E. Von Hipple, "Successful Products from Customer Ideas," *Journal of Marketing*, January 1978.
22. In "Information Flow in R&D Labs," *Administrative Science Quarterly* 14 (1969), T. Allen and S. Cohen analyze the very high leverage such "gatekeeper" activities can have in R&D organizations.
23. J. Schumpeter, *Capitalism, Socialism and Democracy* (New York: Harper & Row, 1975); and M. Maidique, "Entrepreneurs, Champions, and Technological Innovation," *Sloan Management Review*, Winter 1980, present the classic views and data on champions.
24. D. McClelland, *The Achieving Society* (Princeton: Van Nostrand Press, 1961); and G. Bylinski, *The Innovation Millionaires* (New York: C. Scribner's Sons, 1976) offer some specific and interesting insights on entrepreneurial motives.
25. T. Kidder, *The Soul of a New Machine* (Boston: Little Brown, 1981) refers to this as "playing pinball."
26. E. Tauber, "How Market Research Discourages Major Innovation," *Business Horizons*, June 1974.
27. J.B. Quinn, "Managing Strategies Incrementally," *Omega*, Vol. 10, no. 6 (1982).

Technology Policy in Japanese Firms

Decision-making, Supplier Links, and Technical Goals

Bruce Rubinger

ABSTRACT. *The focus of competition among Japanese firms has shifted to the creation and mastery of advanced technology. To harness technology, an integrated system involving the firm and its key suppliers has been created. Like the widely analyzed* kanban *system, the system for managing technology has been adopted by a majority of leading companies. It enables Japanese firms to systematically identify and evaluate R&D opportunities, to augment internal efforts by assimilation of external progress, and to balance short- and long-term needs. Japanese firms have gained many research efficiencies by honing this decision-support structure. The hallmarks of this decision-support system are described, including the role of the Board of Directors, joint R&D with suppliers, the setting of research priorities, and the origins of manufacturing technologies. This structure is illustrated by examining the practices of the Toyota Motor Company, one of Japan's leading high-tech companies.*

During the more than 30 years that Japanese industry was absorbed with catching up to its Western counterparts, it emphasized technology acquisition, productivity gains, and improved quality. By honing the manufacturing system, Japanese firms set new standards for quality while emerging as the low-cost producers. With these manufacturing objectives achieved, they have shifted the focus of competition to the creation and mastery of advanced technology.

While the transition from imitation to innovation has received some publicity in the West, the depth of this commitment is much greater than commonly believed. The perception of technology as a strategic variable is pervasive in Japanese industry. An integrated system involving the firm and its key suppliers has been created to support the management of technology. Like its widely analyzed counterpart, the *kanban* system for enhancing operational performance, the system for manag-

Bruce Rubinger's background is a blend of technology and the science of decision-making. He has devoted the past nine years to analyzing evolving patterns of international competition in technology-intensive sectors. This work has addressed such issues as research and development, international strategic planning, and accelerating information exchange between the US and Japan. Dr. Rubinger is currently the Director of Studies with the Global Competitiveness Council, an independent, Boston-based "think tank." In this position, he is responsible for developing advanced management tools and analyzing international technical trends.

ing technology has been adopted by a majority of leading companies. Since high-tech firms, such as NEC, Canon, Toyota and Mitsubishi, have adopted similar approaches, it is possible to describe their management of R&D by examining the practices of one company. (This article relied heavily on Japanese sources, since there is very little available in the Western literature.)

Toyota As a High-Technology Company

While Toyota's manufacturing expertise has received considerable attention, its R&D activities have been ignored. In fact, very little analysis has been carried out regarding the approach of the Japanese auto industry to R&D management, or the competitive implications of the current research thrust.

This lack of information is unfortunate, since the Japanese auto industry has served as a technology-driver for the Japanese economy. It continues to play this pivotal role as a producer and consumer of advanced technology as Japan's industrial structure evolves toward high technology. For instance, the auto industry currently consumes 10% of all integrated circuits and 20% of all robots.

Toyota Motor Company is actually a high-technology firm, as measured by traditional indices. For instance, during the early 1980s, Toyota had the largest R&D budget of any Japanese firm, though it yielded this position to Hitachi in 1984 (R&D spending by top Japanese firms is illustrated in Table 1). With aggregate expenditures of 190 billion yen in fiscal year 1984, Toyota's R&D budget greatly exceeds that of Toshiba, Fujitsu or Matsushita, firms widely acknowledged as technical leaders in intensely competitive high-tech sectors.[1]

This emphasis on advanced technology is underscored by a breakdown of the high-tech ratio of an automobile (see Table 2). Despite the industry's traditional caution toward the adoption of new technology, an attitude shaped by the severe operational and low-maintenance environment in which cars must operate, advanced technology already represents 32.4% of the cost of an automobile.[2]

TABLE 1. TOP JAPANESE FIRMS IN R & D SPENDING (FY 1984)

RANK	FIRM	EXPENDITURES*
1	Hitachi	210
2	Toyota Motor	190
3	NEC	190
4	Toshiba	150
5	Nissan Motor	150
6	Fujitsu	120
7	Matsushita	120
8	Honda Motor	106
9	Mitsubishi	90
10	Mazda Motor	75

*R&D Expenditures are in billions of yen.
Source: *Japan Economic Journal*, pg. 5, June 26, 1984.

Table 2 THE HIGH-TECH RATIO OF AN AUTOMOBILE
(Toyota Mark II, 2000cc, twin cam)

High-tech part	Added value of high-tech part (unit: 10,000 yen)
Electronically-controlled automatic transmission:	9.9
Electronically-controlled suspension 4-wheel, ventilated disc brakes Speed-sensing power-steering DOHC engine • Computer-controlled system • Variable-induction system	30.9
Electronic skid control:	6.7
Electronic, digital display instrument panel:	4.5
High-grade, body-contoured seats Fully-automatic air conditioner Automatic lighting-control system Automatic power door lock with key reminder	33.0
Total of high-tech parts (A):	85.0
Retail price of the car (B):	262.0
High-tech ratio: (A/B, in %):	32.4

Source: "The Japanese Auto Industry: Active In Research & Development," pg. 3; LTCB Research, Monthly Economic Review, Jan/Feb. 1985.

Toyota also excels at the management of technology. A recent poll of 500 top business executives in Japan ranked Toyota number one for all-around management ability.[3] The factors considered included technical development ability, ability to respond to change, and efficient use of technical personnel. (The ranking of Japanese firms for all-around management ability is presented in Figure 1, and the evaluation criteria appear in Figure 2.) As a result of its ability to balance the requirements of technical innovation with "bottom line" performance, Toyota has emerged as a technological leader, and is reported to be the most profitable Japanese corporation listed on the Tokyo Stock Exchange.[4]

Toyota's research activities are intended to yield a new generation of engines, electrical components, and materials. The firm's extensive progress is evident in Figure 3, "Toyota's Technological Innovations." These innovations include Toyota Electronic Suspension, speak monitor, a fiber-optics-based wiring system, and several new materials used in engine components — heat-resistant alloys, fine ceramics, fiber-reinforced plastics, and engineering plastics. Current specialty applications of new materials are intended to provide vital production experience. The firm anticipates greatly expanded usage of new materials in the future.

Like other Japanese auto producers, Toyota sees tremendous potential from the application of ceramics technology to automobile engine components. Technological advances in this sphere are likely to result in significant commercialization of ceramic engine parts within three years. Likely applications include ceramic pistons, cylinders, precombustion chambers, nozzles, valves, bearings and rotors.[5] Com-

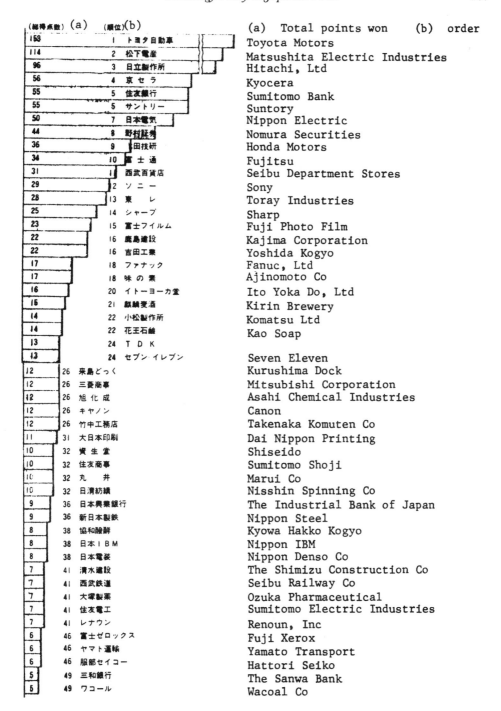

(総得点数) (a)	(順位)(b)		(a) Total points won (b) order
163	1	トヨタ自動車	Toyota Motors
114	2	松下電産	Matsushita Electric Industries
96	3	日立製作所	Hitachi, Ltd
56	4	京セラ	Kyocera
55	5	住友銀行	Sumitomo Bank
55	5	サントリー	Suntory
50	7	日本電気	Nippon Electric
44	8	野村証券	Nomura Securities
36	9	田技研	Honda Motors
34	10	富士通	Fujitsu
31	11	西武百貨店	Seibu Department Stores
29	12	ソニー	Sony
28	13	東レ	Toray Industries
25	14	シャープ	Sharp
23	15	富士フイルム	Fuji Photo Film
22	16	鹿島建設	Kajima Corporation
22	16	吉田工業	Yoshida Kogyo
17	18	ファナック	Fanuc, Ltd
17	18	味の素	Ajinomoto Co
16	20	イトーヨーカ堂	Ito Yoka Do, Ltd
15	21	麒麟麦酒	Kirin Brewery
14	22	小松製作所	Komatsu Ltd
14	22	花王石鹸	Kao Soap
13	24	T D K	
13	24	セブン イレブン	Seven Eleven
12	26	来島どっく	Kurushima Dock
12	26	三菱商事	Mitsubishi Corporation
12	26	旭化成	Asahi Chemical Industries
12	26	キャノン	Canon
12	26	竹中工務店	Takenaka Komuten Co
11	31	大日本印刷	Dai Nippon Printing
10	32	資生堂	Shiseido
10	32	住友商事	Sumitomo Shoji
10	32	丸井	Marui Co
10	32	日清紡績	Nisshin Spinning Co
9	36	日本興業銀行	The Industrial Bank of Japan
9	36	新日本製鉄	Nippon Steel
8	38	協和醗酵	Kyowa Hakko Kogyo
8	38	日本IBM	Nippon IBM
8	38	日本電装	Nippon Denso Co
7	41	清水建設	The Shimizu Construction Co
7	41	西武鉄道	Seibu Railway Co
7	41	大塚製薬	Ozuka Pharmaceutical
7	41	住友電工	Sumitomo Electric Industries
7	41	レナウン	Renoun, Inc
6	46	富士ゼロックス	Fuji Xerox
6	46	ヤマト運輸	Yamato Transport
6	46	服部セイコー	Hattori Seiko
5	49	三和銀行	The Sanwa Bank
5	49	ワコール	Wacoal Co

SOURCE: Leading Industries, Principal Business Executives Rated, "Shukan Daiyamondo," August 13, 1983, in Japanese.

FIGURE 1. Ranking of Japanese enterprises on the basis of all around management ability

Note: The number in the black dot indicates the order

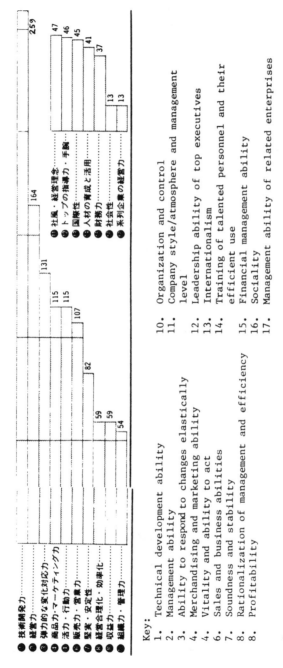

Key:
1. Technical development ability
2. Management ability
3. Ability to respond to changes elastically
4. Merchandising and marketing ability
4. Vitality and ability to act
6. Sales and business abilities
7. Soundness and stability
8. Rationalization of management and efficiency
8. Profitability
10. Organization and control
11. Company style/atmosphere and management level
12. Leadership ability of top executives
13. Internationalism
14. Training of talented personnel and their efficient use
15. Financial management ability
16. Sociality
17. Management ability of related enterprises

[Keyed numbers correspond to numbers in black dots]

SOURCE: Leading Industries, Principal Business Executives Rated, "Shukan Daiyamondo." August 13, 1983, in Japanese.

FIGURE 2. Factors weighed in ranking the management ability of Japanese firms

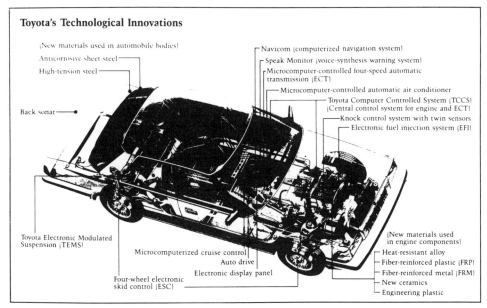

Toyota's Technological Innovations

(New materials used in automobile bodies)
Anticorrosive sheet steel
High-tension steel
Back sonar

Navicom (computerized navigation system)
Speak Monitor (voice-synthesis warning system)
Microcomputer-controlled four-speed automatic transmission (ECT)
Microcomputer-controlled automatic air conditioner
Toyota Computer Controlled System (TCCS) (Central control system for engine and ECT)
Knock control system with twin sensors
Electronic fuel injection system (EFI)

Toyota Electronic Modulated Suspension (TEMS)
Microcomputerized cruise control
Auto drive
Electronic display panel
Four-wheel electronic skid control (ESC)

(New materials used in engine components)
Heat-resistant alloy
Fiber-reinforced plastic (FRP)
Fiber-reinforced metal (FRM)
New ceramics
Engineering plastic

Technological innovations that have been incorporated in the Crown and other Toyota cars are illustrated here on the Crown.

Source: 1983 Toyota Annual Report

FIGURE 3. Toyota's technological innovations

mercial introduction of a ceramic engine by the mid-1990s is anticipated by some industry insiders.

Toyota's transformation into a high-technology firm closely mirrors the restructuring of the Japanese economy toward higher value-added products.[6] In addition to new materials, anticipated advances in the areas of processing, fabrication and assembling, CAD/CAM/CAE, and software engineering systems will provide the foundation for Japan's future competitiveness, according to a survey of "Leading Industrial Technologies of the 1990s."[7] Toyota is a major player in each of these areas.[8] A company with strong national identity, Toyota is committed to playing a major role in achieving Japan's vision as a technology-based nation.

Current Research and Development Expenditures

Toyota uses a broad definition of R&D. It includes any step undertaken to improve the performance and energy efficiency of automobiles.[9] Toyota often counts production-related research and certain TQC- (Total Quality Control) related expenditures as R&D costs. Like other Japanese firms, Toyota is rather liberal in its treatment of R&D costs, which are compiled for the purpose of internal accounting and are not required for a public filing of expenditures.

Toyota's R&D expenditures in fiscal year 1983 were 181 billion yen, or 4% of total sales.[10] This figure, however, seriously underrepresents Toyota's R&D capability, since it does not include the extensive outlays made by affiliated automotive suppliers who are members of the Toyota Group.[11] It is common in industrial groups for there to be considerable intra-group cooperative research and technology sharing.[12]

A breakdown of R&D expenditures by the key members of the Toyota Group is provided in Table 3. When these expenditures are included, R&D spending for the Toyota Group companies approaches 250 billion yen, or approximately $1.1 billion. The data in Table 3 illustrates an important characteristic of intra-group R&D, namely the concentration of R&D among the most sophisticated firms. There is a division of labor under which the most advanced technology is developed for the group by Toyota and a few of its key suppliers, primarily Nippondenso and Aisin Seiki. The R&D activities of the remaining suppliers are oriented toward process technology to attain the quality improvement and cost reduction goals specified by Toyota.

For the purpose of comparison with US R&D expenditures, the above-mentioned R&D figure must be substantially increased for two reasons. First, technology is transferred from the subcontractors to the Toyota parent company at artificially low prices. This is particularly true for the volume of technical information transmitted to the parent corporation during proposal writing stages and for the low price paid by the parent company for the production of innovative technology developed by a group company or subcontractor.

The second factor is the comparatively low cost of conducting R&D in Japan. This reflects the lower salaries paid to technical personnel, since R&D is a very labor-intensive process. For example, the starting annual salary for an engineer in Japan is around $13,000. Other factors contributing to the lower cost of R&D include the reduced cost of capital and research efficiencies achieved by the swift adoption of laboratory automation systems.

TABLE 3. R&D EXPENDITURES BY PRINCIPAL MEMBERS OF THE TOYOTA GROUP FISCAL YEAR 1983*

Company	R&D Expenditures**
Aisin Industry	2,100
Aisin Seiki	9,100
Daihatsu Motor	8,400
Hino Motors	6,600+
Nippondenso	37,300
Toyoda Gosei	3,900
Toyota Motor Company	181,000
Toyoda Machine Works	1,600
Total Group R&D	249,900

*Source: *Kaisha shikiho* 181 (Autumn 1983)
**In million yen
+Estimated by GCC based on sales/R&D ratio for similar firms.

R&D Forecast

Toyota's commitment to heavy R&D spending is expected to continue unabated over the next decade. The firm recognizes that its success lies in providing additional value-added to each automobile, and exploiting new fields on the peripheries of the auto business. Toyota is well positioned to pursue this thrust. The firm's war chest is so substantial that it is often referred to as the "Toyota Bank" by industry insiders. Our projection for future R&D spending is as follows: [13]

Fiscal Year 1982	173 billion yen
Fiscal Year 1983	181 billion yen
Fiscal Year 1984	190 billion yen
Fiscal Year 1985	210 billion yen
Fiscal Year 1986	230 billion yen

Personnel Issues

Approximately 8,000 individuals, 14% of total employees, work in an R&D capacity at Toyota. These employees are normally recruited directly out of universities and have backgrounds in science or engineering.

The company's job rotation pattern means that a high percentage of employees who work in R&D are assigned to positions outside of the technology-related divisions. The company's philosophy places a premium on shop-floor experience. At any particular time, about 35% of the R&D staff is likely to be working in Toyota's production facilities.[14] Job rotation patterns are such that 70% of all engineers will eventually revert back to R&D positions after having been exposed to factory jobs.

R&D personnel receive no special benefits or privileges to foster individual creativity. In fact, individual "geniuses" are actually discouraged. Like other Japanese auto firms, Toyota is acutely aware that, in the future, major technical advances will involve interdisciplinary efforts. "This means that cooperation between different specialties or different industries is necessary for the development of such technologies to meet diverse needs."[15] The firm's emphasis on job rotation and group-oriented research efforts foster interdisciplinary R&D.

Following Japanese tradition, the salaries of R&D personnel are initially determined by their seniority in the company. After a period of ten years, however, the researchers' annual bonus—comprising about 40% of their salaries—is linked to performance. The R&D personnel we interviewed indicated that they are motivated primarily by their sense of contributing to the company, and are less concerned about financial remuneration. There is a strong emotional link to the company and to the individual's small field group.[16] Through company policies that foster intense competition between groups, these sentiments serve as a major source of research vitality.

An important motivating factor for R&D personnel is rank and promotion. R&D engineers participate in regular study sessions and classes designed to advance their technical competence. The engineers' progress is partially measured by their performance on periodic evaluation tests given by Toyota's personnel department. There are numerous grades for the various types of technical positions within the company based on test results and on-the-job performance (*e.g.*, senior engineer). The grades are closely associated with promotions and — perhaps more importantly — recognition within the company. This system of technical rankings and internal recognition is believed by insiders to be instrumental in allowing the company to effectively marshal its engineering resources behind its objectives.

Overall Approach to R&D

Toyota's approach to R&D management involves several critical underlying elements, namely, the role of suppliers, the setting of research priorities, the dividing line between basic and applied research, and the origin of manufacturing technologies.

Joint Activities with Suppliers

Like other major Japanese firms, Toyota typically carries out joint R&D with its parts suppliers. The level of joint research activities between automobile manufacturers and parts producers is considerably higher in Japan than in the US. It encompasses both sophisticated components and low technology items that are referred to as "black box parts." Examples of this joint development are described by Tomisawa.[17]

The extensive reliance on joint development is partly a function of the complex, semi-exclusive subcontractor relationships existing between assemblers and parts manufacturers. In some instances, these links go back more than 30 years. While Toyota does have a large R&D effort in-house, these activities are complemented to a considerable degree by those of subcontractor firms.

Pattern of Joint Activities

The supplier enters into a collaborative relationship with Toyota very early in the product development schedule. The supplier usually assists in the writing of basic specifications during a phase termed "The Concept Study/Product Planning Stage."[18] It is important to note that Toyota will usually seek input from more than one of its preferred subcontractors at this time. This practice permits Toyota to obtain more information and to assure that it receives the lowest bid.

This approach also transfers a significant amount of total R&D cost to the subcontractor. The auto parts industry believes that the drawback of these costs is outweighed by their more stable relationships with assemblers. In addition, parts suppliers are able to determine more efficiently whether a particular R&D activity will lead to commercialization.

Preparation of Proposals

A major function of the suppliers within the Toyota Group is to present the parent firm with proposals for new parts or for improvements in function and specifications of existing parts. Toyota screens and evaluates proposals presented by each supplier.

Finally, decisions on whether to continue basic development work on the part or proceed with the production of prototypes are arrived at through close consultation with the supplier firm.

Strategic Factors in Joint R&D Work

A significant amount of the R&D for new auto parts is conducted independently by the parts suppliers. This holds particularly true for non-strategic parts, such as shock absorbers, headlights, internal accessories, and mass-produced components, such as sparkplugs. Toyota will typically provide detailed information on the parts' performance specifications, cost and interface requirements to these suppliers of "black box components."

In contrast, Toyota and its key suppliers cooperate closely in the development of strategically sensitive parts, notably engine, transmission, and electronic control-related parts. There are two basic reasons for dividing R&D work according to the strategic value of the component in question. First, Toyota believes that technology yields a strategic advantage only if it is proprietary. To protect its corporate investment in R,D&E, it entrusts the development of such strategic parts to only a select few of its leading parts suppliers. The two prime recipients of this trust are Nippondenso and Aisin Seiki.

The second consideration is that R&D in these cutting-edge areas requires extensive technological and financial resources. This has led to the concentration of R&D activity within the Toyota Group, and emergence of a cadre of technically advanced suppliers. The technical capabilities of these first-tier suppliers are widely perceived to be greater than those of their US counterparts. This evolution of R&D capability within the Toyota Group reflects a similar trend underway in Japanese industry at large.

Rationalization and Further Cost Reduction

In contrast to their US counterparts, Japanese manufacturers have an intimate knowledge of the manufacturing costs of their suppliers. This has enabled them to systematically set cost-reduction goals. For instance, in the early 1980s, the car makers demanded that their subcontractors lower break-even volumes, and achieve annual cost reductions of 3–5%. These pressures led to a reorganization of the first-tier parts manufacturers, and the promotion of self supply.[19] The announced price reduction goal for 1985 is more modest—0.5–1.0%—reflecting the fact that the system's efficiency has already been extensively honed through value engineering.

Detailed, Highly Reliable Documentation

Toyota requires extensive documentation from its parts suppliers during the process of presenting proposals for new parts or novel manufacturing approaches. This documentation is provided directly to R&D planning chiefs. While the flow of documentation implies a great deal of trust between the parts supplier and Toyota, it is also true that Toyota's suppliers are resigned to a certain amount of technology transfer via Toyota to another member of the Toyota Group.

Transfer of Data to Third Parties

Because Toyota has a policy of multiple sourcing, it will sometimes provide technology that was developed jointly with one supplier to other suppliers. Conversely, "materials and parts manufacturers which develop a product jointly with one automaker sometimes sell the product to other automakers, too. Often an automaker prohibits the sale of a jointly developed product to other car makers for some fixed period of time, such as a year, with sales unrestricted thereafter."[20]

Personnel Exchange

The process of joint development between Toyota and its group parts suppliers is facilitated by exchange of technical and product planning personnel. Personnel move in both directions: from Toyota to the parts supplier, and vice versa. Time spent by the exchanged engineer at his new workplace ranges from periods of several months to as long as three to five years. Engineers from parts firms sent to Toyota often work with engineers from other parts firms. In some instances, Toyota will suggest that certain of its parts suppliers cooperate in R&D for a particular area.

Research Priorities and Trends

Setting of Basic Research Priorities

Toyota's proposals for R&D originate mainly from its Product Planning Section, the Development Planning Section, and the Product Quality Department of the Research and Development Division (see Figure 4). Proposals regarding vehicle performance, safety, and emissions control come from the Higashi-Fuji Technical Center, which is part of the larger Research and Development Division. Proposals for basic research, which in some cases may not be of immediate use in automotive applications, largely come from the Toyota Central Research and Development Laboratories, Inc., which serves as a sort of "think tank" for the Toyota Group as a whole. Finally, as discussed above, a considerable number of proposals originate from Toyota's major parts suppliers.

Basic Research Areas Supported

Basic research concentrates on the development and application of new materials. Particular emphasis is placed on heat-resistant alloys, fiber-reinforced plastics (FRP), fiber-reinforced metals (FRM), fine ceramics and engineering plastics for engine applications. For example, Toyota became the first automotive firm to successfully develop a FRM for use in steel inserts for piston heads. This work was carried out in conjunction with Art Metal Manufacturing, its affiliated supplier of pistons and piston rings. Development of FRP and FRM for body applications is receiving considerable attention as well. The commitment to ceramic auto parts is also quite extensive. In 1985, the company began production of a ceramic prechamber for its Crown diesel engine.

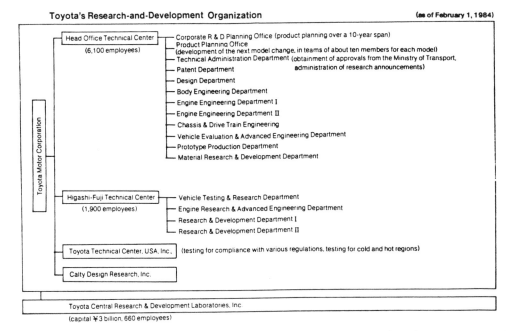

Source: The Japanese Auto Industry: Active in Research and Development," p. 6
LTCB Research, Monthly Economic Review, Jan./Feb. 1985

FIGURE 4. Toyota's research and development organization

Applied Research Areas Supported

Toyota's applied research focuses on automotive electronics, in particular, applications in running safety, engine and power train controls, display communications, and other convenience and comfort items. For instance, in cooperation with Nippondenso, Toyota has developed the first microcomputer-controlled suspension system. The company is strengthening its research activities related to communications, fiber optics, IC manufacturing, and information systems in anticipation of entering those fields.[21] Toyota is also actively pursuing the creation of a new generation of automotive engines, and is conducting applied research in the related areas of combustion, sensors and tribology. This work has led to the commercialization of Toyota's innovative Lean Combustion Engine, which yields a 22% improvement in automobile fuel economy.[22]

To ensure compatibility among the numerous manufacturing systems within the firm and its affiliated suppliers, system integration is another active topic. For instance, Toyota's Central Research and Development Laboratory recently developed an advanced factory robot programming language, "TL-10." By achieving close integration of manufacturing systems within the Toyota Group, the firm will gain further reductions in product launch time.

Dividing Line Between Research and Commercialization

At Toyota—and other Japanese firms, as well—there is a definite trend toward separating the R&D sections which engage in basic research from those responsible for product planning and commercialization. This is a significant departure from the traditional practice of grouping all R&D activities together. The separation between basic and applied research is reflected in the organizational structure. For instance, the Number One Engine Department of Toyota's R&D Division engages in basic engine technology research, while the Number Two Engine Department is more concerned with commercial applications. Regular rotation of personnel between the basic and applied research sections ensures coordination of efforts.

Manufacturing Technology

Toyota's policy is to develop all significant manufacturing technology in-house. It is summarized by Chairman Eiji Toyoda's precept, "Intuition is developed through repeated practice. Once developed, there is an accumulation of past knowledge, and answers emerge naturally without requiring new information."[23] Thus, the expertise essential for identifying future process improvements and assuring close integration between process and product technology can only be gained through the in-house creation of manufacturing technology.

Toyota has made great strides in introducing robotics and larger factory automation systems over the past few years, spurred on by arch-rival Nissan's automated Zama factory. Its original focus was on painting, welding and assembly robots. In 1985, the emphasis shifted to the introduction of flexible manufacturing systems into its engine, transmission and body welding lines. This flexibility will enable the company to spur sales by providing customers with a greater variety of options.

The overall pattern followed by Toyota is to purchase industrial robots and other automation hardware from outside suppliers and to develop the software in-house. The Production Technology Division plays a pivotal role in coordinating production automation activities and planning future programs.

Organizational Structure

The organizational structure of Toyota's R&D effort involves two major divisions, several technical research centers, subsidiaries and captive parts firms. The two main divisions are the Research and Development Division and the Product Technology Division.

Research and Development Division

Toyota's R&D organization is illustrated in Figure 4. Each division is headed by a senior manager who is also a director of the company. Below the divisions are departments, such as the Prototype Production Department or the Number One Engine Engineering Department. These operations are headed by department heads, called *bucho* in Japanese. These individuals, about 45 years old, are usually concerned with the administrative management of their respective departments. The implementation of research activities, including the submission of research proposals, is the responsibility of section head managers, *kacho*, who tend to be about 35 years old.

Production Technology Division

The Production Technology Division employs about 7,400 people, and its organization roughly parallels that of the R&D Division. It includes the "Production Engineering Development Department which plans how to improve production through flexible manufacturing systems and robots, the Production Engineering Planning Staff Office, which plans how to change which production lines at the various factories, the Engineering Department, which is in charge of developing technology for various phases of manufacturing, such as assembly, presses, welding, painting and forging, and the Machine Tool Manufacturing Department, which develops and manufactures machine tools."[24]

Toyota Central Research and Development Labs

The research labs consist of six divisions, employing some 800 researchers. Their purpose is to conduct "fundamental research for the Toyota Group." The labs have an annual budget of 10 billion yen ($39.8 million), of which 80% is devoted to research on topics suggested by Toyota Group companies, while the remainder addresses longer-term research issues.

Decision Structure

Toyota has developed a sophisticated decision process for setting research directions and balancing its short- and long-term R&D requirements. This structure is best illustrated by the examination of procedures for establishing research policy and evaluating the merits of individual projects.

Research Policy

Technology policy is established at the top of the corporation by the Board of Directors. This approach is supported by the inclusion of the senior R&D managers on the board. In addition, the use of a tight system of progress reports allows senior managers to closely monitor technical activities within the firm. After a revised corporate technology policy is formulated, it is widely discussed by corporate staffers and suppliers. Following a typical Japanese management pattern, the solutions are then formulated at the bottom of the organization and passed up through the chain of command.[25]

Another distinctive aspect of R&D at Toyota is that the Board of Directors will periodically initiate research efforts. This role ensures the necessary support for long-term activities essential to the future competitiveness of the firm. Long-term research is thereby insulated from the tough hurdles which ordinary research projects must pass.

Project Initiation and Review

The screening of R&D proposals is the responsibility of the section heads. The most attractive proposals are then forwarded to the department heads for review and approval. Proposed projects that survive this scrutiny are forwarded to committees composed of directors and division chiefs. For any major R&D undertaking, the approval of the Board of Directors will also be required.

Once a project is initiated, a Design Chief is appointed. His job is to coordinate activities with the different departments and outside suppliers. These slots are usually filled by senior engineers. Another key mechanism for ensuring close communication among employees is the design review. Toyota conducts design reviews at five different stages. For instance, the planning design review is intended to prevent the recurrence of problems encountered in previous models, and occurs prior to prototype planning. At the prototype stage design review, models are evaluated on the basis of CAD drawings and other technical information to confirm that they perform according to the specs.

During the design reviews, progress will be compared against that of other competing projects. The review committee will cancel a program if it feels that other developments within Toyota or affiliated firms or changes in market conditions rule out the need for the project. Industry insiders estimate that the percentage of R&D proposals which result in new parts or components is less than 5%. This figure is considerably lower than that for comparable US firms. The low success rate reflects the large number of competing R&D proposals within the Toyota Group. It is not a symptom of R&D inefficiency, but rather a characteristic of a vigorous, highly focused process.

Conclusions

Technology plays an increasingly central role in the competitive strategy of Japanese firms. To harness technology, they have created an integrated decision structure involving the firm and its key suppliers. Hallmarks include extensive communication among the entire employee community during all phases of the R&D process; establishment of long-term goals by the Board of Directors; and intense intra-firm competition. This system enables Japanese firms to systematically identify and evaluate R&D opportunities, augment internal efforts by assimilation of external progress, closely couple R&D to market needs, and balance short- and long-term needs.

Japanese firms have gained many research efficiencies by honing the decision-support infrastructure. This has led to a division of labor within the group which creates first-tier suppliers that are among the world's most technologically advanced. Both strong and weak members of the group benefit from the synergies. In contrast, the management of technology in US firms is still often the responsibility of a small group of managers and researchers and possibly a few internal entrepreneurs. Given the critical role of technology, US firms should not continue to marshal their technological resources solely in this manner. Where appropriate, US firms should learn from the experience of effective Japanese companies like Toyota, and begin to expand the involvement and scope of R&D in the corporation in a determined, comprehensive and strategic fashion.

Acknowledgment

The author wishes to thank Dr. Susan Weiner, Manager of the Council's Japan Desk, for her survey of Japanese R&D information and translation of key materials.

Notes

1. "Corporate R&D Spending Continues to Grow Sharply," *Japan Economic Journal*, June 26, 1984, p. 1. For R&D spending in the early 1980s, see "Japan's Role in Revitalizing World Industry," *The Wheel Extended*, March 1983.
2. Konomi Tomisawa, "The Japanese Auto Industry: Active in Research and Development," *Monthly Economic Review*, LTCB Research, January–February 1985.
3. "Leading Industries, Principal Business Executives Rated," *Shukan daiyamondo*, August 13, 1983 (in Japanese).
4. In 1984 profits hit a new record of Y527 billion ($2.1 billion), or more than twice that of the second most profitable firm. See "Pretax Recurring Profits of 11 Automakers," *The Japan Economic Journal*, May 7, 1985, p. 20.
5. M. Kono, "Status and Problems of Fine Ceramics," *Tsusansho koho*, January 28, 1984, pp. 5–11 (in Japanese).
6. For a description of the Japanese economy's high-tech transformation, see *Japan Economic Almanac 1985*, pp. 65–111 (Nihon Keizai Shimbun, Inc., publisher).
7. "Leading Industrial Technologies of the 1990s: Survey by the Industrial Technology and Economic Research Institute," reported in *Shukan daiyamondo*, August 1983 (in Japanese).
8. See "R&D Unit Pursues Non-Auto, High-Tech Products," *The Japan Economic Journal*, July 9, 1985, p. 7; and Toyota Motor Company Annual Report 1984.
9. As in the US, the definition of R&D expenditures (*Kenkyu kaihatsu hi*) is quite broad. According to the authoritative R&D source, *Nikkei shakai joho* (p. 986), it is defined as "expenses related to the development of new products or new processes. The standard Japanese definition comes from Section 36 of the Financial Statements Regulation. Since it is amortized in the appropriate period, it includes personnel expenses. However, there are cases where companies define R&D expense in their own unique way. This includes instances when the method of calculation follows the tax deduction criteria of exceptions to the Tax Laws Act. That definition includes expenses for materials, personnel, depreciation of facilities and buildings, and technology licensing fees, but excludes the cost of land and interest."
10. Fiscal Year 1983, ending in March 1984, is the last year for which complete R&D data for the firm and its affiliated suppliers is available.
11. For a description of the Toyota Group, see "Industrial Groupings in Japan, 1984–1985," Dodwell Marketing Consultants, Tokyo, Japan; and Toyota Motor Company Annual Report 1984, p. 45.
12. See "Intra-Group Cooperation Enhanced in High Technology R&D and Other Fields," *The Japan Economic Almanac 1985*, p. 215.
13. To accurately describe investment trends, all R&D data is given in yen. The conversion rate on July 15, 1985, was 237 yen to the dollar.
14. "Emphasizing the Worker at the Jobsite," interview with Dr. Shoichiro Toyoda, President, Toyota Motor Company, in *The Wheel Extended*, Vol XIV, no. 1 (1984), pp. 12–18.
15. S. Ohigashi, "Japanese Technology in the 1990s," *JSAE Review*, March 13, 1984, p. 5.
16. For a discussion of field-groups and the individual's emotional ties to a company, see N. Yamaki, "Social Climate and Management Practice in Japan," *Management Japan*, Vol. XVII, no. 1 (Spring 1984), pp. 7–17.
17. Tomisawa, *op. cit.*, pp. 7–8.
18. *Jidosha no kihon keikaku to dezain* (Product Planning and Engineering of Automobiles), 1980, translated by T. Fujimoto.
19. "Progress of Technological Innovation in the Japanese Machine Industry and Subcontract Manufacturers," *Engineering Industries of Japan*, no. 22 (June 1982).
20. Tomisawa, *op. cit.*, p. 8.
21. "R&D Unit Pursues Non-Auto, High-Tech Products," *op. cit.*
22. "Development of the Toyota Lean Combustion System," *JSAE Review*, July 1984, pp. 106–111.
23. "Seeing Things As They Are: The Starting Point for Production," interview with Eiji Toyoda, *The Wheel Extended*, Vol. XIV, no. 1 (1984), p. 6–11.
24. Tomisawa, *op. cit.*, p. 8.
25. A. Oozuka, "Japanese Business Leaders: How Do They Rise to the Top?," *The Wheel Extended*, Vol. XI, no. 4 (October–December 1981).

Executive Succession, Strategic Reorientations, and Organization Evolution

The Minicomputer Industry As a Case in Point

Michael L. Tushman, Beverly Virany and Elaine Romanelli

ABSTRACT. *This longitudinal study investigates the determinants and effects of executive succession for high- and low-performing minicomputer organizations. Findings suggest that performance shortfalls drive executive succession in low performers, while strategic reorientations prompt succession for high-performing firms. The effects of succession depend on whether strategic reorientation accompanies executive change. Only when executive succession occurs with reorientations does future organization performance increase. Otherwise, there is no association between executive succession and subsequent organization performance. Executive succession and strategic reorientation appear to be important strategic levers affecting organizational performance over time.*

Effective top-level leadership has long been recognized as a critical component of corporate strategy (Barnard, 1938; Selznick, 1957; Andrews, 1980). Moreover, the enormous impact of the chief executive officer (CEO) or equivalent in modern high-technology industries has also been documented (Freiberger and Swaine, 1984; Malone, 1985). Executive leadership is particularly critical in technology-based organizations because shifts in product and/or process technologies have an enormous impact on bases of competition. Changes in product class conditions require

Michael L. Tushman is a Professor of Management at the Graduate School of Business, Columbia University. He has a B.S.E.E. from Northeastern University, an M.S. from Cornell University, and a Ph.D. from MIT, the latter two degrees in Organization Studies. His research and consulting center on those strategic and organizational factors affecting the performance of technology-based organizations. Professor Tushman lectures throughout the United States, as well as in Japan and throughout Europe.

Beverly Virany is a Doctoral Candidate in Management of Organizations at Columbia University. She has a B.S. in Economics from the Wharton School of the University of Pennsylvania. Her research focuses on examining management teams and their impact on corporate strategic behavior.

Elaine Romanelli is Assistant Professor of Organizational Behavior at the Fuqua School of Business, Duke University. Her research focuses on strategies and processes of new venture formation. She has published articles in Management Science *and* Research in Organizational Behavior. *She received her Ph.D. in Management of Organizations from Columbia University.*

different kinds of competence in an executive team, and may require fundamentally different organization forms (*e.g.*, Lawrence and Dyer, 1983).

At least part of the reason for substantial organization decline in the face of environmental change lies with the executive team. A set of executives who have been historically successful may become complacent with existing systems and/or be less vigilant to environmental changes. Or, even if an executive team registers external threat, they may not have the energy and/or competence to effectively deal with fundamentally different competitive conditions. The importance of an effective executive team is accentuated in industries where the rate of change in underlying technologies is substantial (*e.g.*, Chandler, 1962; Quinn, 1981).

Given the importance of the executive team in managing their organizations as competitive conditions change, this article investigates the determinants and effects of executive succession on a cohort of firms in the minicomputer industry. It explores factors which affect executive succession and conditions under which executive succession is associated with increased organization effectiveness. We find that both executive succession and strategic reorientation are important levers in keeping organizations aligned with changing environmental conditions.

Background and Hypotheses

Building on a long history of work on organization evolution (*e.g.*, Norman, [1977]; Miller and Friesen, [1984]), Tushman and Romanelli (1985) argue that organizations evolve through periods of relative equilibrium, punctuated by strategic reorientations. Reorientations are sharp discontinuities in the life of a firm in that they involve simultaneous shifts throughout the organization (*e.g.*, in strategy, power, structure and controls). Strategic reorientations end one convergent period and, in turn, begin the next convergent period. Quite different than reorientations, convergent periods are characterized by incremental change to refine and further bolster an existing strategic orientation.

This punctuated equilibrium approach to organization evolution focuses on periods in the life of an organization (or business unit) and on the role of reorientations in redirecting organizations under crisis conditions and/or as product-class conditions change. Where organizations are constrained by social and structural inertial forces, strategic reorientations are an important mechanism by which organizations can realign themselves with environmental demands.

Executive leadership (that is, the CEO and his/her top team) plays a critical role in mediating between environmental forces for change and internal forces for stability. Only they can initiate, shape and direct reorientations. The paradox, however, is that while strategic reorientations must be initiated by executive leadership, the same inertial processes which dampen organizational responsiveness also affect executive leadership's ability to attend to and deal with environmental change. Inertial processes reduce the probability that executives will vigilantly attend to or accurately process shifts in environmental conditions. Even if environmental threat is registered, the response of highly inertial systems to external threat is frequently increased reliance on traditional response patterns (Staw *et al.*, 1981; Kiesler and Sproull, 1982).

The more historically successful and/or older the organization, the more tradition and precedent operate to insulate executive leadership from environmental shifts (Boswell, 1973; Hall, 1976). These inertial processes are further accentuated the more homogeneous the executive leadership team, the greater its tenure, and the greater its degree of ownership (Allen and Panian, 1982; Katz, 1980; Wagner *et al.*, 1984). Given these inertial processes and rigid response patterns associated with high threat conditions, Tushman and Romanelli (1985) hypothesize that strategic reorientations will occur most frequently under crisis conditions, and will be most frequently driven by a new set of executives hired from outside the organization (see also McEachern, 1975; Gordon and Rosen, 1981; Pfeffer and Salancik, 1978). While existing executive leadership is not precluded from implementing reorientations, such occurrences are exceptions.

This metamorphosis model of organization evolution with its emphasis on environmental change, convergent periods punctuated by discontinuous change, and on the critical role of executive leadership, provides a foundation for hypotheses on determinants and effects of executive succession.

Determinants of Executive Succession

If there is a consistent result in the executive succession literature, it is that poor organizational performance is a major determinant of executive succession. In times of poor performance, executives are likely to be replaced (James and Soref, 1981; Allen *et al.*, 1979). A firm's performance and the associated performance of the executive team is likely to be judged based on changes relative to the organization's past performance.

> *Hypothesis 1:* Organization performance change will be negatively associated with executive succession.

Strategic reorientations are transformational events which involve discontinuous changes throughout the organization. Given commitments existing managers have to prior courses of action, reorientations will be associated with executive succession (Carlson, 1961; Helmich and Brown, 1972). While existing managers are not precluded from implementing reorientations, such occurrences will be exceptions. Reorientations will be most likely initiated by externally recruited executives (Gordon and Rosen, 1981; McEachern, 1975).

> *Hypothesis 2:* Strategic reorientations will be positively associated with executive succession.

Discontinuities in product-class conditions change the nature of competition within the product class. For example, in the minicomputer industry, the advent of semiconductor memory (1971–72) and the advent of microprocessors (1975–77) each transformed the nature of the product, its served market and related production processes (Tushman and Anderson, 1985). Legal, political and/or social discontinuities (*e.g.*, deregulation or oil crisis) also affect bases of competition within a product class (*e.g.*, Miles, 1982).

Environmental discontinuities create fresh demands on an executive team built on previous environmental opportunities and constraints. For example, after chip technology was developed, the basis of competition within the minicomputer niche shifted from technological sophistication to marketing responsiveness (Fishman, 1982). One way organizations can keep current with changing competitive conditions is through executive succession. Newly hired and/or promoted executives may possess more current information about competitively important demands (*e.g.*, Pfeffer and Salancik, 1978).

Hypothesis 3: Environmental discontinuities will be associated with increased executive succession.

Organization inertia is accentuated the more insulated the executive team is from its environment because of ownership conditions (Allen and Panian, 1982). Organizations which are closely held by management are less coupled to environmental conditions than organizations that are widely held. Closely held firms are more susceptible to idiosyncratic demands of the executive team, and are less likely to initiate changes in the executive team than widely held firms. The other extreme occurs when a concentrated amount of a firm's stock is held in outsider's hands. In such situations, management's insulation is stripped and executives are more open to opposition (James and Soref, 1981; Allen, 1981).

Hypothesis 4: The greater the degree of management ownership, the less the executive succession.

Hypothesis 4A: The more externally controlled the organization, the greater the degree of executive succession.

Effects of Executive Succession

Three contradictory viewpoints exist on the effects of executive succession on subsequent organizational performance. Gouldner (1954) and Grusky (1960) found that executive succession was negatively related to organizational outcomes. Grusky (1964) and Allen *et al.* (1979) found this negative relation accentuated when managers were recruited from outside. Guest (1962) and Helmich (1974), however, found a positive relation between executive succession and organization performance, while Gamson and Scotch (1964) found executive succession unrelated to subsequent organization performance.

These contradictory results indicate that executive succession is a disruptive event which by itself may not be associated with subsequent organization effectiveness. Executive succession by itself may be smothered by organization inertia and/or by managerial resistance to change (*e.g.*, Hall, 1976). However, if executive succession is coupled with strategic reorientations, the combination of leadership changes and system-wide organization changes may break the grip of organization inertia and add needed executive energy and competence. Under crisis conditions and/or when environmental conditions change, executive succession coupled with reorientation may increase survival odds when compared to studied inaction or inaction due to tentative change resisted by internal forces for stability (see Figure 1).

Hypothesis 5: There will be no association between executive succession and subsequent organization performance.

Hypothesis 6: The combination of executive succession with strategic reorientations will be positively associated with subsequent organization performance.

Succession Patterns for Historically High and Low Performing Firms

The metamorphosis model of convergence and reorientation provides insight into the manner in which historically high performing firms evolve as compared with low performers. Such distinction builds on the paradoxical character of convergent periods. In one respect, inertial processes operating during convergent periods hinder the organization's ability to reassess environmental opportunities. On the other hand, the stability of convergent periods facilitates organizational learning and coordination. In contrast, reorientations and major executive changes are disruptive, risky and costly to undergo. High performing firms avoid the disruptive consequences of overly frequent successions and reorientations and capitalize on the benefits of convergent periods. Rather than avoiding executive change entirely, high performers are expected to experience executive succession primarily when faced with major environmental discontinuity. Such environmental changes provoke the need for new executive expertise to help reorient the organization to fit its evolving environment.

Hypothesis 7A: High-performing firms will have a history of fewer executive succession events than low-performing firms.

Hypothesis 7B: For high-performing firms, major succession events which do occur will correspond to environmental discontinuities and/or reorientations. Performance shortfalls will be less of a driving force for high-performing firms as compared with low performers.

Sample and Methods

This research employs a cohort-based longitudinal design. All minicomputer firms born between 1968–1971 (N = 59) were identified (excluding firms which only added peripherals and/or software to another firm's minicomputer). Table 1 provides a list of these firms. Data on each firm was gathered on a year-by-year basis from its birth through 1980 (or until it failed or was acquired). These data were gathered from 10-K's, annual reports, industry journals, and business press, and via interviews with industry experts. Detailed succession data were available for 37 firms. Because data were not available on firms that entered and immediately exited the niche, our sample is biased towards those firms which survived at least two years. Our sample includes firms with substantial variability in organization performance and fate.

Executive Succession: The degree of executive succession was measured on an annual basis for each firm. In determining the degree of executive succession, we distin-

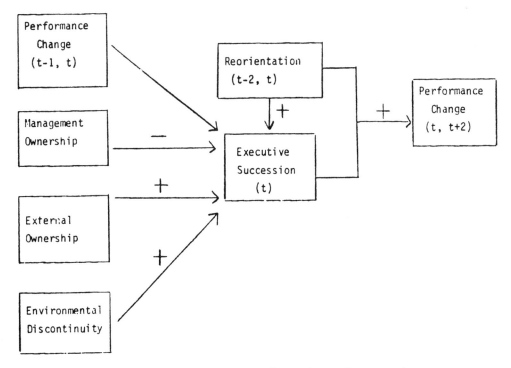

FIGURE 1. Determinants and effects of executive succession.

TABLE 1. Minicomputer firms born between 1967–1971

Artronix	Educomp/Quodata	Minuteman Computer Corp.
Atron Inc.	Eldorado Electrodata	Modular Computer Corp.
Business Controls Corp.	Electronic Processors	Monitor Data
California Data Processors	Foto-Mem Inc.	Multidata
Cascade Data Computers	Four-Phase Systems	Northwest Data Systems
Compiler Systems	General Automation	Omnus Computer Corp.
Computer Automation	GRI Computer Corp.	Peripherals Interface
Computer Communications	Hetra Computers &	Prime Computers
Computer Development	Communications	Qantel Corp.
Computer Interactions	Imlac	Rolm Corp.
Computer Logic Systems	Incoterm	Spiras Systems
Computer Signal Processors	Information Technology	STC Systems
Comstar	International Computing Co.	Sycor Inc.
Data 100	Interplex	Systems Computer Corp.
Datacraft	Linolex	Tempo
Data General	Martin-Wolfe Inc.	Unicom
Datapoint	Megadata	Unicomp
Decade Computers	Microdata	Varisystems
Digital Computer Controls	Micro Systems Inc.	Viatron
Digital Scientific	Mini Computer Systems Inc.	Wilkinson Computer Sciences

guish between the following continuum of possibilities ranging from no succession to major succession:

NO CHANGE   0 = no senior executive change
    1 = change in senior executive (below CEO)
    2 = change in CEO, where such successor is an insider
MAJOR CHANGE 3 = change in CEO, where such successor is externally re-
    cruited

An individual was classified as a senior executive if that person is of the highest rank (based on title) immediately below the CEO. Two types of executives were considered senior: (1) the president, where a different individual was listed as CEO, and (2) an executive or senior VP in firms which designate individuals as such.

The classification of CEO varied depending on the manner in which firms listed their officers. The CEO was considered either: the Chairman of the Board (unless the chairman was listed as an outsider with other full-time responsibilities), the CEO, or the president (in cases where no other individual is listed as Chairman or CEO). A successor is deemed externally recruited if he or she held a position outside the organization less than one year prior to the appointment; otherwise, the succeeding executive is classified as an insider.

Retirement of executive officers is not relevant for this sample of firms. The average executive age was 40. Of the 396 executives studied, only four were older than 60. Given the relative youth of executives in this cohort, executive age is not used as an explanatory variable in predicting executive succession.

Reorientations: Reorientations are systemic, organization-wide changes defined here by simultaneous changes in strategy, power, structure and controls. Histories of each firm were gathered to empirically identify the existence of reorientations. To obtain this range of organizational data, detailed year-by-year data were gathered on each firm in the cohort. These data were gathered from 10-K's, prospecti, annual reports, industry reports, market research reports, and industry publications, and from business press. Data were gathered and coded by different researchers to minimize bias.

Strategy changed if either the firm's core product line changed or its served markets changed; power changed if resources devoted to functional areas shifted dramatically and/or if power changes were discussed in the business/industry publications; structure changed if the firm's core structural form changed; and control changed if content analysis of annual reports and/or industry publications indicated changes in technical and/or social modes of control.

Data on changes in strategy, power, structure and control were gathered on a year-by-year basis for each firm. Reorientations are those events where strategy, power, structure and controls all change concurrently. Because reorientations occurred over two-year periods, reorientations were coded as "1" if strategy, power, structure and controls *all* changed over a two-year period; otherwise reorientation was coded as "0" for those years. For those firms (N = 4) where annual reports were not available, reorientations were coded as "1" if strategy and two other core variables changed over a two-year period. Three independent coders consistently identified over 85% of the reorientations. Discrepancies were discussed, and remaining reorientations coded.

Ownership and Control: Both internal and external ownership variables were considered. Internal ownership was measured by the percentage of common stock held by management. This includes aggregate holdings of the CEO and executive team. External ownership was measured as the percentage of common stock owned by the largest outside shareholder. These data were obtained from firm 10-K, annual reports, and industry sources.

Performance: Performance and performance change were measured by return on assets (ROA) on a yearly basis. Firms in the sample were classified as historically high performers by comparing firm ROA to industry average ROA. Firms were categorized as high performers if their ROA was greater than industry average ROA for all years—excluding the firm's start-up period, and allowing for at most one outlier year of low performance later in the company's life (16 firms were so categorized). Organizations were classified as low performers if their ROA was below industry average for the majority of years of their operation (seven firms were so categorized). Organizations which did not meet either performance criterion were dropped from those analyses comparing high vs. low performing organizations.

Results

Determinants of Executive Succession

Table 2 (Column A) displays the simple correlation between degree of executive succession and ROA change measured one year prior to succession. The data sup-

**TABLE 2. Correlations between degree of executive succession
and change in firm performance[1]**

Variable	(A) Full Sample	(B) High Performers	(C) Low Performers
ROA change— 1 year prior to succession	−.28***	.009	−.50***

***$p \leq .005$

[1]The following is pertinent to Tables 2–5:

Number of observations range between:
117–219—for full sample correlations
29–136—for high performers' correlations
6–43 —for low performers' correlations
(only 1 correlation with n < 20)

ports Hypothesis 1, demonstrating a significant inverse relationship between performance change and executive succession. Although not shown on Table 1, a similar analysis using market share growth was also performed. While the significance of the result is weakened when utilizing a market share measure, the direction of the relationship is consistent with those reported in Table 2. Performance decline is significantly associated with increased executive succession.

Hypothesis 2 argued that there would be a positive association between strategic reorientations and executive succession, that new executives are required to implement system-wide changes associated with reorientations. Because of the time lag between reorientations and executive team change, reorientations were associated with executive succession if they occurred within a two-year period prior to succession. The correlations in Table 3 (Column A) support Hypothesis 2; there is a significant positive relationship between reorientations and executive succession. Supporting these data, the mean amount of executive succession is more than two times greater during reorientations than during convergent periods (.70 vs. .27; $p < .01$). Evidently, major executive changes are often made to implement reorientations.

Hypothesis 3 suggested that executive succession would be an instrument for organizations to attend to and deal with environmental discontinuities. Our expectation was that the discontinuous price/performance consequences of semiconductor memory (introduced between 1971–72) and microprocessors (introduced between 1975–77) would affect the bases of competition within the minicomputer product class, and, in turn, be associated with greater executive succession. The time span under study, 1968–1980, was segmented into five periods: 1968–70; 1971–72; 1973–74; 1975–77; 1978–80. A one-way analysis of variance was used to test for differences in the mean amount of succession between time periods. There were no significant differences in executive succession between periods ($F = .75$; $p = .56$). We find no support for our hypothesis that the degree of succession is higher during periods of sharp technological change.

Simple correlations in Table 4 (Column A) provide insight on Hypotheses 4 and 4A. Hypothesis 4 — predicting a negative relationship between the amount a firm is closely held by management and succession — does not gain support. No significant correlation is found between the amount of common stock held by the firm's management and the degree of executive succession. There is support, however, for Hypothesis 4A. There is a significant positive correlation between the degree the firm is externally controlled and major succession events. It appears that powerful

TABLE 3. Correlations between degree of executive succession and reorientations

Variable	(A) Full Sample	(B) High Performers	(C) Low Performers
Reorientations	.16**	.20**	.34**

**$p \leq .05$

TABLE 4. Correlations between degree of executive succession
and ownership variables

Variable	(A) Full Sample	(B) High Performers	(C) Low Performers
Percent Common Stock Owned by Management	.12	− .02	− .08
Percent Common Stock Owned by Largest Outsider	.26***	.10	.54***

***p ≤ .005

outside owners show their opposition to existing top management by having them removed from office.

Multiple regression was used to explore the relative strengths of performance change, reorientation and ownership on executive succession (see Table 5). Size (as measured by number of employees) was added into the regression equation as a control variable (see James and Soref, 1981). Consistent with results above, the regression indicates that executive succession is driven by performance decline and the initiation of reorientations. External ownership has no independent impact on succession. Organization size is inversely associated with executive succession. The significant negative relationship of number of employees is interesting given Grusky's (1961) argument that large firms are more prone to top succession. In contrast the negative relationship found here further supports an inertia argument. Larger organizations are more inertial, making executive change more difficult to

TABLE 5. Regression results on determinants of executive succession

	ROA Change (t-1, t)	Size	External ownership	Reorientation (t-2, t)	R^2	d.f.
A. Full Sample	− .48**	− .00005**	.003	.24**	.16	118
B. High Performing Organizations	− .11	− .00003	.005	.24*	.08	83
C. Low Performing Organizations	− .62*	− .00003	.01	.45	.47	16

*p < .005
**p < .025

accomplish. The regression coefficients indicate that organization size is, however, a much weaker determinant of executive succession than either performance change or reorientation.

Effects of Executive Succession

Table 6 (Column A) provides insight on effects of succession (Hypotheses 5 and 6). Table 6 (Column A) presents correlations between the degree of executive succession and subsequent firm performance (ROA growth measured two years following the succession event). Data is provided for the sample as a whole, as well as for two subgroups: (1) observations during years in which reorientations occurred, and (2) remaining observations during which reorientations did *not* occur.

Hypothesis 5 suggested that there would be no direct association between executive succession and subsequent change in performance. Hypothesis 6 argued that the combination of executive succession and reorientations would be positively associated with performance change. Contrary to Hypothesis 5, data in Table 6A indicate that there is a significant positive correlation between executive succession and subsequent organization performance. Consistent with Hypothesis 6, however, the positive association between succession and subsequent performance holds only when succession occurs with reorientations. When successions occur without reorientations, there is no association between succession and subsequent performance. These data provide insight into the conditions under which executive succession is associated with increased organization effectiveness. It is only the combination of succession with reorientation that results in enhanced effectiveness. Succession and reorientation by themselves are not associated with increased organization effectiveness (the correlation between reorientation and subsequent performance is $-.04$; $p = .60$).

Succession Patterns for Historically High and Low Performing Organizations

The remaining results focus on succession patterns for historically high- and low-performing organizations. In support of Hypothesis 7A, historically high-performing

TABLE 6. Correlations between degree of executive succession
and subsequent performance[1] under varying conditions

	(A)	(B)	(C)
Conditions	Full Sample	High Performers	Low Performers
Unconditional	.18**	.26***	.27
Reorientation	.43***	.51***	.50
No Reorientation	.02	.13	.05

$**p \leq .05$
$***p \leq .005$
[1]Subsequent performance—ROA change measured 2 years following the succession measurement

organizations have significantly less executive succession than low-performing organizations (.19 vs. .72; p < .01). Indeed, low performing organizations have more than three times the amount of executive succession than high-performing organizations. Where high-performing organizations have the same average number of reorientations as historically low performing organizations ($\bar{x}$ = .24), high performing organizations are able to implement these system-wide changes with a relatively small amount of executive succession.

A closer examination of succession events for high-performing firms reveals two distinct patterns. Six of the 16 high-performing firms had no executive succession over the entire period studied. Those high-performing firms without executive succession initiated as many reorientations as the other high-performing firms, but they did so without executive succession. These extraordinary firms were able to break up prior inertial periods and implement reorientations without changes in the executive team. On the other hand, the other high-performing firms did not have significantly less executive succession than all other firms in the cohort. These high-performing firms engaged in major executive succession to accomplish all reorientations.

The set of high-performing firms without executive succession were exceptional, not only in their succession/reorientation patterns, but in their performance records as well. These six firms were the largest and fastest growing firms in the cohort. Table 7 demonstrates that these firms had both significantly greater absolute sales and market share growth than the other high performing firms. The historical success of these firms may in part be attributable to their unusual ability to reorient while maintaining greater executive team stability (Tushman and Romanelli, 1985). Thus, Hypothesis 7A is partially supported. Of the high-performing firms, one set had no executive succession; the other set of high-performing firms had as much executive succession as other firms in the cohort.

Hypothesis 7B argued that the determinants of executive succession would be different for historically high vs. low performing organizations. We argued that environmental discontinuities and reorientations would drive executive succession for historically high performing organizations, while performance decline would drive executive succession for historically low performing organizations.

TABLE 7. Comparing high-performing firms

	No Executive Change (n = 6)	With Executive Change (n = 10)	Difference Between Means
Mean Reorientations	.24	.25	not significant
Mean Sales	3815	1810	***
Mean Sales Growth (measured over 2 years)	1945	1008	***

```
  * = p < .05
 ** = p < .01
*** = p < .001
```

Years with environmental discontinuities had no more executive succession events than years without environmental discontinuities for both high- and low-performing organizations (F = 1.36, p = .25 and F = 1.5, p = .22 for high- and low-performing firms, respectively). Evidently technological discontinuities by themselves are not immediately associated with executive succession. There is a positive association between reorientation and executive succession for both high- and low-performing organizations (see Table 3). In support of Hypothesis 7B, performance change is negatively associated with executive succession only for low-performing organizations. Where high-performing organizations did have decreases in ROA over the years studied, these decreases were not associated with executive succession (see Table 2).

While no hypotheses were offered on the relationship between ownership patterns and succession for high and low performing organizations, these data are reported in Table 4. The only significant correlation is between the degree the firm is externally controlled and executive succession for low-performing organizations. For high-performing organizations, ownership conditions have no association with executive succession. Outside shareholders exercise their power to provoke major executive succession for low performing organizations, however. Managerial ownership is unrelated to executive succession for both high and low performing organizations.

What are the relative strengths of performance change, reorientation, and external ownership in explaining executive succession for high- and low-performing organizations? Table 5 presents separate multiple regressions exploring the determinants of executive succession for historically high- and low-performing organizations. In support of Hypothesis 7B, the comparative regressions demonstrate quite different primary forces driving executive succession for high- and low-performing organizations. Where ROA change is the only significant predictor of executive succession for low-performing organizations, reorientation is the only significant predictor for high-performing organizations.

These data provide support for Hypothesis 7B. Executive succession for high-performing organizations is driven by strategic reorientations. Neither performance change nor environmental conditions affect executive succession for high-performing organizations. For low-performing organizations, however, executive succession is driven primarily by declining performance. Neither reorientation nor environmental conditions nor ownership conditions had a significant independent association with executive succession for low-performing organizations.

These data provide insight into the conditions under which historically high- and low-performing organizations initiate executive succession. High-performing organizations seem to initiate executive succession in order to implement strategic reorientations. Linking succession and reorientation is a positive maneuver for these firms to maintain their successful competitive position as market conditions evolve. Low-performing organizations, on the other hand, recruit new executives when faced with performance-related crises. These two scenarios illustrate the widely different conditions under which successors in high- vs. low-performing organizations assume responsibility. Such differences are likely to impact the manner in which the new executives implement change. Note that the most effective firms in this cohort initiated as many reorientations as other firms, but with no executive succession. The historical success of these few extraordinary organizations may be in part attributed to their ability to reorient while maintaining executive team stability.

To what extent are the consequences of executive succession different for historically high- vs. low-performing organizations? Table 6 presents correlations between executive succession and subsequent performance for high- vs. low-performing organizations. These data indicate that there are no differences in the succession-subsequent performance linkage between high- and low-performing organizations. As with the full sample, executive succession is only associated with subsequent performance if succession is linked with reorientations. Executive succession without reorientation is not associated with future performance under any conditions. (The absence of a significant relationship for the low-performing group is due to the small number of observations where low-performing organizations initiated reorientations ([N = 6]).

Discussion

Executive leadership mediates between internal forces for stability and external forces for change. As environmental conditions change, the importance of executive leadership is accentuated in that organizations must attend to and deal with competitive opportunities and threats. Building on a metamorphosis approach to organization evolution, this research has explored both determinants and effects of executive succession. Executive succession and strategic reorientations seem to be important strategic levers affecting organization performance over time.

Performance decline and strategic reorientations are important determinants of executive succession; each are associated with increased executive succession. The relative impact of these factors is different for high- vs. low-performing organizations. For high-performing organizations, reorientations were the single most powerful predictor of executive succession. High-performing organizations may initiate executive succession in order to successfully implement proactive reorientations. For low-performing organizations, however, performance decline is the dominant factor driving executive succession. Low-performing organizations bring in new executives in order to stem declining performance.

Major environmental change, seen here as technological discontinuities, was not related to concurrent succession events. It may be that environmental shifts are related to executive succession over time. As environmental discontinuities do affect bases of competition (*e.g.*, Tushman and Anderson, 1985), future research could investigate the time lags between environmental shocks and executive succession. Ownership patterns did not have a major impact on executive succession. The greater the external ownership of a firm, however, the greater the degree of executive succession for low-performing organizations. Evidently, outside owners exert control under poor performance conditions.

The determinants of executive succession are quite different for historically high- vs. low-performing organizations. High-performing organizations initiate executive succession to implement strategic reorientations, while low-performing firms initiate executive succession under crisis conditions. High performing organizations seem to utilize new executives to implement proactive reorientations (that is, re-orientations prior to performance decline). Low-performing organizations, on the other hand, bring in new executives to turn around organizations in crisis.

Historically high-performing organizations had significantly less executive succession than low-performing organizations. There were two types of succession patterns identified for high-performing organizations. The most successful high-performing organizations had no senior executive or CEO succession. These visionary executives implemented proactive reorientations with a stable set of senior managers. The other high-performing organizations had the same overall amount of executive succession as other organizations in the cohort. These high-performing organizations utilized executive succession as a vehicle to initiate and implement proactive strategic reorientations.

Those high-performing organizations with no top executive change were far and away the most successful firms in the cohort. These extraordinary firms initiated as many reorientations as other firms, while maintaining the existing senior management team. While the vast majority of reorientations are implemented with sweeping changes in the executive team, it may be that the minority of reorientations driven by the same top executives are the most effective — resulting in the historical success of this extraordinary set of organizations. Future research could explore the nature and characteristics of such visionary executive teams which initiate vast organizational changes prior to organization decline.

Neither reorientations nor executive succession, by themselves, were associated with enhanced organization performance. Only when executive succession was coupled with reorientation did subsequent performance increase. These patterns were found for both high and low performing organizations. Evidently, the impact of executive succession by itself is smothered by entrenched forces for stability, while reorientation without executive succession is resisted by an unwilling (or incapable) executive team. It is the combination of executive succession with reorientations which simultaneously breaks organizational inertia and provides a fresh set of executives to implement organization-wide changes.

Coupling executive succession with reorientations may be the kind of maneuver to insure the continued success of high-performing organizations which face changing competitive conditions, and the kind of aggressive action required to turn around organizations in crisis. Those most extraordinary firms, however, initiated proactive reorientations with no senior executive succession. These organizations were able to take advantage of stability in the executive team in implementing reorientations to take early advantage of competitive opportunities. Future research could provide greater clarity on the conditions under which executive succession is associated with future organization effectiveness.

The cohort nature of this research has many advantages in that it tracks a set of firms, born at the same time, and competing in the same markets, over a 14-year period. This research design, however, clearly suffers from limited external validity. Future research could utilize cohort based designs on other industries. Such programmatic research would provide data on intra- and inter-industry determinants and consequences of executive succession.

Conclusion

As competitive conditions change, fundamentally different organization forms are required. However, due to organization inertia, many organizations either do not effectively attend to environmental change or, if the threat is registered, act to bolster the status quo. This research indicates that both executive succession and strategic reorientations are important strategic levers affecting organization evolution. Those most effective organizations initiated proactive reorientations with no top executive succession. Visionary CEO's are rare indeed. Other high-performing organizations initiated proactive reorientations along with major executive changes. The combination of executive changes along with organization-wide changes were associated with increased organization effectiveness. Historically low-performing organizations, however, tended to initiate executive succession under crisis conditions. As with high-performing organizations, coupling executive succession with reorientation was associated with enhanced organization effectiveness. Where executive succession and reorientations are by themselves not associated with increased organization performance, when linked together they have a strong positive effect on subsequent performance.

Executive succession and strategic reorientations are important factors affecting organization effectiveness over time. Future research must extend our knowledge of the determinants and effects of executive succession, and broaden our knowledge on the timing and linkages between executive succession, strategic reorientations, and environmental conditions.

Acknowledgments

The authors would like to thank Phil Anderson, Robert Drazin, and Don Hambrick for their advice and encouragement. The Strategy Research Center, Graduate School of Business, Columbia University, provided support for this research.

References

Allen, M.P., "Managerial Power and Tenure in the Large Corporation," *Social Forces* 60 (1981), pp. 482–494.
Allen, M.P., S.K. Panian and R.E. Lotz, "Managerial Succession and Organizational Performance: A Recalcitrant Problem Revisited," *Administrative Science Quarterly* 24 (1979), pp. 167–180.
Andrews, K.R., *The Concept of Corporate Strategy* (Homewood, IL: Irwin, 1980).
Barnard, C.I., *Functions of the Executive* (Cambridge, MA: Harvard University Press, 1938).
Boswell, J., *The Rise and Fall of Small Firms* (London: Allen & Unwin, 1973).
Carlson, R.O., "Succession and Performance Among School Superintendents," *Administrative Science Quarterly* 6 (1961), pp. 210–227.
Carroll, G.R., "Dynamics of Publisher Succession in Newspaper Organizations," *Administrative Science Quarterly* 29 (1984), pp. 93–113.
Chandler, A., *Strategy and Structure* (Cambridge, MA: MIT Press, 1962).
Eitzen, R. and N. Yetman, "Managerial Change, Longevity, and Organizational Effectiveness," *Administrative Science Quarterly* 17 (1972), pp. 110–116.
Fishman, D., *The Computer Establishment* (New York: Harper & Row, 1982).
Freiberger, P. and M. Swaine, *Fire in the Valley* (Berkeley, CA: Osborne/McGraw-Hill, 1984).
Gamson, W. and N. Scotch, "Scapegoating in Baseball," *American Journal of Sociology* 70 (1964), pp. 69–76.
Gordon, G.E. and N. Rosen, "Critical Factors in Leadership Succession," *Organizational Behavior and Human Performance* 27 (1981), pp. 227–254.
Gouldner, A.W., *Patterns of Industrial Bureaucracy* (New York: Free Press, 1954).

Grusky, O., "Administrative Succession in Formal Organizations," *Social Forces* 39 (1960), pp. 105–115.

Grusky, O., "Corporate Size, Bureaucraticization, and Managerial Succession," *American Journal of Sociology* (1961), pp. 261–269.

Grusky, O., "Managerial Succession," *American Journal of Sociology* 49 (1963), pp. 21–31.

Grusky, O., "Reply to Scapegoating in Baseball," *American Journal of Sociology* 70 (1964), pp. 72–76.

Guest, R.H., "Managerial Succession in Complex Organizations," *American Journal of Sociology* 68 (1962), pp. 47–54.

Hall, R.H., "A System Pathology of an Organization: The Rise and Fall of the Old Saturday Evening Post," *Administrative Science Quarterly* 21 (1976), pp. 185–211.

Helmich, D.L., "Organizational Growth and Succession Patterns," *Academy of Management Journal* 17 (1974), pp. 771–775.

Helmich, D.L. and W.B. Brown, "Successor Type and Organizational Change in the Corporate Enterprise," *Administrative Science Quarterly* 17 (1972), pp. 371–381.

James, D.R. and M. Soref, "Profit Constraints on Managerial Autonomy: Managerial Theory and the Unmaking of the Corporate President," *American Sociological Review* 46 (1981), pp. 1–18.

Katz, R., "The Effects of Group Longevity on Project Communication and Performance," *Administrative Science Quarterly* 27 (1982), pp. 81–104.

Kiesler, S. and L. Sproull, "Managerial Response to Changing Environments: Perspectives on Problem Sensing from Social Cognition," *Administrative Science Quarterly* 27 (1982), pp. 548–570.

Lawrence, P. and D. Dyer, *Renewing American Industry* (New York: Free Press, 1983).

Malone, M.S., *The Big Score: The Billion Dollar Story of Silicon Valley* (Garden City, NY: Doubleday, 1985).

McEachern, W.A., *Managerial Control and Performance* (Lexington, MA: D.C. Heath, 1975).

Miller, D. and H. Friesen, *Organizations: A Quantum View* (Englewood Cliffs, NJ: Prentice Hall, 1984).

Normann, R., *Management for Growth* (New York: Wiley & Sons, 1977).

Pfeffer, J. and G.R. Salancik, *The External Control of Organizations: A Resource Dependence Perspective* (New York: Harper & Row, 1978).

Quinn, J.B., *Strategies for Change: Logical Incrementalism* (Homewood, IL: Irwin, 1981).

Romanelli, E. and M.L. Tushman, "A Quasi-Experimental Design Proposal for Longitudinal-Comparative Research," *Management Science* (in press).

Salancik, G.R. and J. Pfeffer, "Effects of Ownership and Performance on Executive Tenure in US Corporations," *Academy of Management Journal* 23 (1980), pp. 653–664.

Selznick, P., *Leadership in Administration* (Evanston, IL: Row, Peterson & Co., 1957).

Staw, B.M., L.E. Sandelands and J.E. Dutton, "Threat-Rigidity Effects in Organizational Behavior: A Multilevel Analysis," *Administrative Science Quarterly* 26 (1981), pp. 501–524.

Stinchcombe, A.L., "Social Structure and Organizations," in J.G. March, ed., *Handbook of Organizations* (Chicago: Rand McNally, 1965).

Tushman, M. and P. Anderson, "Technological Discontinuities and Organizational Environments," Strategy Center Working Paper, Columbia University, 1985.

Tushman, M. and E. Romanelli, "Organizational Evolution: A Metamorphosis Model of Convergence and Reorientation" in L. Cummins and B. Staw, eds., *Research in Organizational Behavior* (Greenwich, CT: JAI Press, 1985).

Wagner, W.G., J. Pfeffer and C.A. O'Reilly III, "Organizational Demography and Turnover in Top Management Groups," *Administrative Science Quarterly* 19 (1984), pp. 74–92.

The Role of Japan-Based R&D in Global Technology Strategy

D. Eleanor Westney
and Kiyonori Sakakibara

ABSTRACT. *For US technology-intensive corporations striving to develop effective global strategies, the establishment of R&D facilities in Japan is increasingly seen as a necessary means of tailoring products to the large local market, of effective technology scanning of Japanese competitors, and of tapping into Japan's growing capabilities in science and technology. The establishment and management of such facilities, however, is no easy task. A comparative study of US and Japanese computer firms identified major differences on five dimensions: the corporate research structure, the linkage between R&D and manufacturing, mechanisms of recruitment of R&D personnel, career patterns and the locus of responsibility for careers, and reward and incentive systems. These differences have important implications for US firms trying to set up research facilities in Japan, both in terms of managing those facilities effectively and in terms of integrating them into the firm's overall technology strategy.*

Global technology strategy has at least two elements: the effective exploitation of the firm's technology in all of the world's major markets, and the utilization and coordination of the technological resources of all the world's "cradles of innovation", not simply those of the home country.[1] For many US firms, accustomed to decades of US dominance of scientific and technical innovation, the transition to a genuinely global technology strategy is a painful process, and nowhere are the difficulties greater than those posed by Japan.

Japan is one of the world's three major markets (the second largest single market after the United States). Yet with some notable exceptions US high technology firms, which are encountering Japanese competitors in the US market as well as in third country markets, have a relatively low level of market penetration there. Both competitor and technology scanning in Japan are therefore comparatively difficult for US firms. Given Japanese technological strengths and the prospects for future

D. Eleanor Westney is Assistant Professor of Management at the Alfred P. Sloan School of Management, MIT, and holder of the Mitsuibishi Career Development Chair in International Management. Her fields of interest include cooperative organizational behavior (with a special focus on Japan) and cross-societal organizational learning.

Kiyonori Sakakibara is Associate Professor of Commerce at Hitotsubashi University in Tokyo and was a Visiting Scholar at MIT in 1984. His major fields of interest are corporate strategy, the management of technology, and internal corporate venturing.

enhancement of those strengths, this is a serious barrier to the development of genuinely global technology strategies.

A growing number of US high technology firms are turning to the establishment of R and D facilities in Japan as a key element of their global competitive strategies. Corning Glass, Digital Equipment, and Teradyne have set up their own research and development facilities in Japan in the past four years; Data-General and Hewlett-Packard have acquired majority ownership of Japanese firms with R&D capabilities. Other firms are considering following suit.

One powerful motive behind the establishment of such research facilities is a growing commitment on the part of major US firms to developing a significant presence in the Japanese market, both because of the sheer size of that market and because of a perceived need for a strategic response to the increasing presence of Japanese competitors in the US domestic market. A research facility in Japan can improve significantly the firm's ability to tailor products to the demands of Japanese customers.

A second and perhaps equally powerful motive is the difficulty of effectively monitoring developments in Japanese science and technology and the technology strategy of Japanese firms from a vantage point in the United States.

Finally, there is growing recognition that Japan is developing comparative advantages in certain areas of technology that can make an important contribution to the technology portfolio of the firm. The perceived success of IBM's subsidiary in Japan, whose research labs have made major contributions to the corporation's worldwide product lines, may also be an incentive for US firms, especially those in the computer industry.[2]

Managing R & D facilities in Japan, and integrating them effectively with the overall technology strategy of the firm is no easy task for a US company. The differences between Japanese and US research organizations are often imperfectly understood, and the management problems can be exacerbated by a lack of strategic coherence in the expectations generated within the firm by the establishment of a Japanese research operation. This article examines the factors behind the growing interest of US high technology firms in developing a research presence in Japan, and draws on the findings of a comparative study on the organization of R&D in Japanese and US computer firms to indicate some of the major problems in effectively pursuing this internationalization of R&D as part of a global technology strategy.

Japan's Growing Technology Resources

In general, large Japanese firms have two major areas of competitive advantage in technology over US firms. First, they have developed ways of embodying technology in products and moving from development through manufacturing to the marketplace quickly, with high quality, and with a relatively low purchase price.[3] Second, Japanese firms have extremely effective systems of global technology scanning, developed over decades of playing "catch-up" in science and technology. These include systems of global patent scanning, in-house international scientific and technical information systems, and high-level technology scanning systems in their foreign subsidiaries. They have been aided in their efforts by the Japanese government, which funded the establishment of a global scientific and technical information system through JICST (the Japan Information Center for Science and Technology), 60% of which covers non-Japanese material.[4] The fact that the Japanese school system provides six years of English language instruction means that most Japanese scientists and engineers have an effective reading knowledge of English and can easily keep abreast of English-language technical publications.[5]

Until very recently, however, the success of Japanese firms at process innovations and the rapid application of technology, and their ability to identify and acquire technical innovations developed in other countries have been widely interpreted abroad as indicative of Japan's inability to innovate.[6] The resulting sense of superiority has meant that US and European firms have been relatively slow to respond to the growing capacity of the Japanese research community with effective scanning systems of their own.

The long-standing image of the Japanese as clever technology imitators but not technology generators, however, is giving way to a recognition of the growing strength of Japanese scientific and technological research capacity. There is both an increased international appreciation of the importance of Japanese process and engineering innovations, and general agreement among technical experts that, in fields such as VLSI, robotics, computers, materials science and engineering, and biotechnology, Japanese researchers are working at the frontiers of existing knowledge.[7] Japan now ranks third in the world, after the USSR and the United States, in the scale of its research capacity, measured either by total expenditures on research or by the total number of active researchers. Scientific and technological research has absorbed a steadily increasing proportion of Japan's expanding national income. The results can be seen in the fact that although Japan still has a deficit in its technology balance of payments, owing to the payment of royalties on long-standing licensing agreements, on new technology agreements Japan has—since the mid-1970s—earned more by selling its technology abroad than it has paid to import technology.[8]

In the coming years, therefore, the significance of the contribution of Japanese researchers is likely to continue to increase, and to move more and more into "state of the art" research. Both Japanese firms and the Japanese government have identified the expansion of the country's basic research capacity as a major priority for the coming decade.[9] The government, with its already high deficits, is somewhat limited in its contribution to this effort. Its rigid restrictions on the acceptance by national universities of outside research funding have been relaxed, and it remains committed to funding research projects in its government labs. However, even when defense expenditures are eliminated from the calculations, direct government contributions to R&D in Japan remain considerably below the levels of the United States and Europe, and are likely to remain so.[10] The major research push is coming from the leading Japanese firms.

The "Limits of Followership"

They are motivated by a belief that Japan is approaching the "limits of followership." Growing resentment of Japanese "technology copying" is producing an increasing reluctance on the part of US and European firms and individuals to license technology to Japanese firms, and greater aggressiveness in pursuing legal redress for perceived infringements on proprietary technology. Even more important is that Japan is—in many areas of science and technology—approaching the limits of existing research, and is itself on the frontiers of knowledge. Large Japanese firms already maintain large central research labs and they are moving in significant numbers to enhance their research capacity. As *Business Week* recently reported, Japanese manufacturers have established more than 25 new industrial research labs during the past two years.[11]

In other words, Japanese firms are moving to add enhanced research capacity to their already impressive capacity for engineering, process and product innovations, and their highly developed systems of global technology scanning. The image of absolute US superiority in science and technology is one which is difficult for many Americans to shed, but there is growing recognition that to keep abreast of important developments in science and technology it is increasingly necessary to monitor Japanese research.[12]

This is not an easy task for US researchers and US firms. Estimates put the amount of Japanese scientific and technical literature that is translated into English at about 25% of the total,[13] and less in some fields. However, even if 25% of published articles find their way into English, this does not mean that 25% of the total body of research is available in English, nor that it is available in timely fashion. Technical translations often leave much to be desired: a translation of a technical article, however well-intentioned the translator, is usually more difficult to follow and less clear in details than the original. There is also a substantial bias in what gets routinely translated. Basic research in scientific journals is more likely to be translated than technical articles in company journals, for example. Translation is expensive, and more important, time-consuming. An additional problem is that getting access to Japanese-language publications within the United States is not easy. The routine acquisition of the flood of Japanese publications in scientific and technical fields is well beyond the resources and perhaps policies of most of the best research libraries.

In addition, experts in some fields have recently noted a new and potentially significant trend: As Japan's own research establishment grows and Japanese researchers have a larger and more sophisticated domestic audience for their research, they seem to be less likely to undergo the difficulties of writing in English and submitting to the laborious review processes necessary to publish in English-language journals. Instead, they can increasingly get useful and speedy feedback by publishing only in Japanese journals.[14]

Moreover, being abreast of published research is only part of the task of keeping up with scientific and technical developments. Few US researchers would rely solely on publications to keep them informed of developments in their field: The informal networks that link researchers are an important part of the scientific and technical information system. Given the explosion in research publication over the last decade, these information networks provide an invaluable guide to what publications are significant, as well as to what research is being carried out prior to the publication stage. Such networks are perhaps even more important in Japan than they are in the United States: Less of the scientific and technical literature is indexed in Japan, and there is a greater tendency to publish in "house organs" of the firm or the university, rather than in nationally refereed journals. The filtering and alerting functions of informal professional networks are therefore extremely important in the Japanese context. Yet comparatively few US researchers have access to such networks within Japan.[15]

Two Dimensions

US firms therefore have strong strategic reasons to develop at least technology scanning facilities in Japan. Such scanning has two dimensions: One is keeping abreast of Japanese developments so as not to have the firm's researchers covering problems already dealt with by their Japanese counterparts; the other is monitoring the technology strategy of major Japanese competitors, a critically important part of effective competitor scanning. The first scanning dimension is most effectively carried out by people who are actively involved in research within the firm: They alone have the expertise to identify what information is of critical importance. In other words, scanning to identify key scientific and technical resources is most effectively carried out by a subunit that itself possesses a research capability.

Still another argument for setting up research facilities in Japan is that in a number of areas the Japanese are developing comparative research advantages that are unlikely to be matched within the United States in the near future. One of these is in materials science and engineering, where the Japanese — driven by their poverty of natural resources and dependence on imported materials — have greater incentives to develop new materials (such as ceramics) than US firms in their comparatively resource-rich environment.[16] Another critical area is the computer and communications field, where Japanese-language processing (with its two 50-character syllabaries and 1780 "everyday use" Chinese characters) makes technical demands that simpler English-language processing does not. The technical solutions to the problems, however, (greatly increased memory, distinctive storage architecture, greater screen definition for monitors, more versatile printers, voice recognition systems for input) have broad applicability to general products. Tapping into the distinctive competence of Japanese research in these areas provides yet another incentive for developing a research presence in Japan in such industries.

In summary, there are four major motivations behind the establishment of R&D facilities in Japan by US high-technology firms: technology scanning to identify scientific and technical research that would be a significant input into the research process of the firm as a whole; technology scanning to analyze the technology strategy of Japanese competitors; research to tailor products to the demands of the Japanese market (particularly important in fields such as computers that demand Japanese-language capability); and research that taps into the comparative advantages of Japanese science and technology to contribute to world-wide product development and the firm's overall technology strategy.

Contrasts in R&D Organization in Japan and the United States

The interest in Japanese management in recent years has produced a considerable body of research on the differences between large US and Japanese firms in terms of the organization and careers of managers and of blue-collar workers.[17] There has been very little comparative study, however, of the organization and careers of research and technical personnel. In 1984, therefore, we carried out a comparative study of the organization and careers of engineers in R&D in three Japanese firms in the computer industry (Fujitsu, NEC, and Toshiba) and three US firms (Data-General, the Digital Equipment Corporation, and Honeywell Information Systems).[18] We were concerned with two critical questions. First, are there aspects of Japanese R&D organization from which US firms would benefit by applying in their own operations? Second, what are the implications for US firms trying to internationalize their R&D strategy by setting up research facilities in Tokyo?

The study identified major differences between the US and Japanese firms on five major dimensions: the corporate research structure and the differentiation of R&D units; the linkage between R&D and manufacturing, especially in the hand-off of research; mechanisms and criteria of recruitment of R&D personnel; career patterns and the locus of responsibility for careers; and reward and incentive systems.

The three Japanese and three US firms are not strictly comparable as firms, but their differences are representative not only of the different structure of the computer industries of the two countries but of the differences in the structure of high technology industries in general.

Each of the Japanese firms is a large, integrated electrical equipment manufacturer, with a broad range of products and a structure that is highly standardized across those product lines. All three Japanese firms were founded before World War II, and the emerging divisions in computers and information systems adopted and adapted existing corporate patterns of R&D. All three Japanese firms have two levels of R&D facilities; corporate-level central research laboratories, and divisional-level R&D units attached to the business divisions, which are centered on manufacturing.

The central research labs conduct basic research and new product development (usually to the stage of the development of the first prototype); the divisional-level research labs carry new product development through manufacturing and testing, carry out research on product enhancement and improvement, and work on improvements in production technology. The firms' desire to maintain the standardization of structures and careers across product lines within these facilities has severely limited the firms' flexibility in developing distinctive career and reward structures in high technology areas. It has led several firms in this industry to set up separate companies in fast-growing and competitive research areas, such as software, to escape from the standardized patterns of the parent firm.

Among the US firms, two are much younger and more specialized than the Japanese firms, and have developed their R&D organization in response to the emerging demands of the industry, and the needs and predilections of the engineers who have dominated it. Even in the case of the third firm, Honeywell, which is part of a huge and highly diversified corporation, the Office Management Systems Division, on which our research was focused, seems to be a fairly autonomous facility that has developed along the same lines as those of its competitors in the industry rather than adapting and integrating with other Honeywell structures.

All three US firms also have two levels of R&D organization, which may at first glance seem to be analogous to the Japanese structures. All three US firms have

Advanced Technology Groups which are working, as the name implies, on new technologies and applications. There are clear differences across the two societies, however. The American Advanced Technology Groups are much smaller than the Japanese central labs, they specialize more in the initial stages of R&D, and they play a less crucial role in new product development.

A Striking Difference

One of the most striking differences between the US and the Japanese firms was that US development and design groups were much less closely linked to manufacturing than their Japanese counterparts, at all levels: the corporate level, in terms of R&D funding and the physical location of research activities; the level of the project group and internal technology transfer; and the level of the individual engineer, in terms of career patterns and significant reference groups.

In the Japanese firms, half the research budget is allocated directly to the central R&D lab, and half is allocated through the business divisions, which can use their funding either to carry out development activities within their own facilities or to commission specific research projects from the central labs. Because of this quasi-market relationship, the business divisions, which in Japan are centered on manufacturing, are, in effect, important internal clients of the central labs. Their power and status within the company as a whole and especially in their interactions with the central R&D lab is therefore very high, especially in comparison to the status of manufacturing in the US firms.

Because the divisions have their own development labs, the handoff of research projects from the central lab to manufacturing takes place at a fairly early stage, often while the formal specifications are still flexible. Engineers in the divisional labs therefore play an important role in the R&D process, and ease of manufacture is a major consideration in the design process. Moreover, the research hand-off is usually accomplished by dispatching one of the engineers from the central lab's project team to the divisional lab. This transfer is permanent, not temporary; it is a step in the engineer's career path, and takes place after he has been with the central lab for six or seven years. It is the first step in a career ladder that leads into line management in the divisions. This contrast with the US firms in terms of the dual career ladder should be noted. In the US firms, the managerial rungs of the dual career ladder led into R&D management; in Japan, they led into line management in the operating divisions.

Internal technology transfer in the Japanese firms seems to follow the maxim that, to move information, you move people. Perhaps because this transfer is standard and expected by the individual engineers, people in the manufacturing are a much more important reference group for central lab engineers than they are for their US counterparts, as Table 1 indicates.

The recruitment of R&D personnel is another aspect of R&D organization on which US and Japanese firms differ dramatically. Recruitment is much more centralized and standardized in the Japanese firms. In our US firms, recruitment was the responsibility of the individual research groups, whose members were heavily involved in the recruitment process. In Japan, recruitment is the responsibility of

TABLE 1. Engineers' reference group

Respondents were asked to select three of the following groups in whose eyes they wished to do well, and to rank order them from 1 (most important) to 3 (third most important). The following table shows the mean ranking for the samples as a whole.

	RANKING Japan (n = 206)	(Mean Score) U.S. (n = 101)	
Research administrator of your group	1 (2.389)	5 (.660)	***
Professional colleagues within your own group	2 (1.320)	1 (2.155)	***
People in Manufacturing divisions	3 (.827)	7 (.112)	***
Top executives in your company	4 (.716)	4 (.730)	***
Professional colleagues elsewhere in your company	5 (.385)	2 (1.005)	***
People in sales/marketing	6 (.216)	8 (.102)	
Respected friends outside your company	7 (.058)	6 (.282)	**
Your family	8 (.053)	3 (.870)	***

***p < 0.001
**p < 0.01

the corporate personnel department; it takes place once a year, and virtually all recruits to the central research labs are new graduates.

These graduates are brought into the firm by highly routinized paths. Key professors in the major Japanese universities routinely allocate their students to the major companies. Although student desires are consulted to some extent, the professor in charge of placement will usually write only one letter of recommendation for each student, and that will be to a major company that will accept without question that recommendation. For a company to disregard the recommendation would be to forfeit the opportunity to obtain future graduates from that professor. For the student to refuse to go to the company for which the professor has written the letter would mean that he would forfeit all chance of working for a major Japanese firm, since the companies do not recruit students for which such letters are not written.

As a result of this system, the leading Japanese companies tend to hire a fixed number of students from the major universities each year. They also make ongoing efforts to establish and maintain close relationships with leading universities through the supply of equipment, research grants to faculty, and personal contacts (for example, personnel staffers frequently visit professors and university placement officers). The lower-ranking universities have a less secure place in the technical job market, and professorial recommendations do not carry nearly the same weight with companies. For graduates of such universities, companies are more inclined to make hiring decisions on the basis of an assessment of the engineer's quality (an assessment assisted by a rigorous written technical exam).

The transfer of engineers from the central labs to the divisional labs is an example of the third major contrast between the Japanese and US firms: the standardization of career patterns. The US engineers and personnel managers we interviewed scoffed at the idea of describing a "typical" career in R&D in their firm. The frequent mobility across firms, the extent of individual options for pursuing new specialities through outside study, the level of individual choice in moving across projects—all these factors make it difficult to describe a "typical" career.

Japanese engineers and managers, on the other hand, had no hesitation in describing the "typical" career for an engineer who joined the central research labs. He (and it was invariably a "he"; to date, no women have been hired as engineers in the central labs of the three Japanese firms) would be recruited directly from university, usually with a master's degree. None of the three companies had any established mechanism for recruiting mid-career engineers, and they said it was very rare for them to do so.

The fact that recruitment takes place once a year allows the companies to put each year's hires through an introductory training program that includes both technical and managerial recruits. This program introduces the recruits to the company, exposes them to the range of functions, and provides them with an intense, shared experience that establishes the basis for horizontal communication after they have dispersed to their new positions.

The engineer whose new position is in the central research lab would spend the first two years in the central labs on a succession of projects, largely in an apprenticeship role. In all three companies, research managers estimated that it took two years before an engineer was capable of making an independent contribution to the research process. He would become more and more active on a succession of projects over the next four to five years, and then would be transferred to the divisional labs, usually as the principal carrier of a research project on which he had taken the major role. Very few engineers remain for their entire careers in the central labs.

As one might gather from the recruitment patterns and from the earlier discussion of career paths within the firm, in the US firms, the locus of responsibility for the engineer's career lies unquestionably with the individual; in the Japanese firms, it lies with the firm. To give one example, the questionnaire respondents in the US firms cited their own expressed wishes as the most important factor in the assignment to their last research project; for Japanese engineers, it was the supervisor of their previous project (see Table 2).

The same pattern could be seen in responses to a question about the motives for taking technical courses since graduation (see Table 3).

Japanese engineers were much more likely to have been assigned to the course by the company; US engineers were much more likely to take the course to improve their career opportunities.

The standardization of careers in Japan extends even to the area of rewards and incentives. In contrast to US firms, where outstanding performance is quickly rewarded with salary increases and promotions, personnel managers in all three Japanese firms insisted that neither salary nor rapid promotion were used to reward exceptional performance. Even the most brilliant engineer proceeded up the salary ladder at the same pace as his peers. The principal rewards for outstanding performance were intrinsic (the respect of superiors and peers) and long-term (the opportunity to go abroad for advanced study, for example, and the prospect of staying in the central lab rather than transferring to the divisions).

TABLE 2. Factors in assignment to last project

Question: "In your assignment to your last project, how much influence did each of the following have in your getting that assignment?

NOTE: Mean score of 5-point, Likert scale from 1 = very little influence to 5 = very great influence.

	Mean		
	Japan (n = 202)	U.S. (n = 95)	t
Your previous supervisor	4.44	2.77	***
Manager of your department / job	3.44	2.62	***
Head of your project	3.92	3.07	***
Personnel staff	1.47	1.35	
Your own expressed wishes	2.94	3.90	***

***p < 0.001

The standardization of Japanese career paths is accentuated by the fact that the organizational structure of the R&D groups is the same as that of manufacturing or sales: the hierarchy of sections (*ka*) and departments (*bu*) is identical, and the titles of section chief and department head carry the same status in every function. They also carry much the same salary across functions.

This standardization of careers and rewards is part of the difference between the two sets of firms in the factors that influence promotion to project leader, although other factors are also involved. Our US respondents rated "technical expertise" as the most important factor in being promoted to project leader; it ranked fourth of five factors for the Japanese respondents. This reflects an important difference in the role of the project leader. In the US firms, the project leader is expected to be a technical leader, who has won his position and commands respect by virtue of his

TABLE 3. Comparison of motives for taking courses

Question: "How important was each of the following motives for taking these courses?

Motives	Mean		
	Japan (n = 123)	U.S. (n = 55)	t
To update existing skills	4.10	4.07	
To add new skills	3.98	4.58	***
To improve chances of promotion	2.02	2.70	***
To improve chances of assignment to more interesting activities	2.35	3.08	***
Assigned to course by company	3.17	1.30	***

(1) Mean score of 5-point, Likert scale from 1 = unimportant to 5 = very important.
(2) *** indicates a t-test with probability p < 0.01

TABLE 4. **Important factors in the promotion to project leader**

Question: "What factors do you think are the most important in being promoted to project leader in your company?"

NOTE: Mean score of importance (3 points for the most important factor, 2 points for the second, 1 point for the third, and 0 point for others).

	Japan (n = 206)		U.S. (n = 103)	
	Mean	(Ranking)	Mean	(Ranking)
Seniority***	1.36	(2)	0.66	(4)
Track record of participation in successful projects	1.42	(1)	1.67	(2)
Administrative ability***	1.27	(3)	0.52	(5)
Technical expertise***	1.17	(4)	1.81	(1)
Ability to work well with others***	0.74	(5)	1.48	(3)

***p < 0.001

mastery of engineering and his ability to find solutions to problems. In the Japanese firms, his seniority has much more importance, and his role is more that of the effective chairman, encouraging and guiding his research team. In both sets of firms, as we can see from Table 4, a track record of participation in successful projects is seen as very important.

But our interviews confirm the fact that such a track record indicates different things in the two contexts. In the United States, it is an indicator of technical mastery; in Japan, it is an indicator of the ability to manage a team successfully.

Four of these five areas of difference—linkage with manufacturing, recruitment, career patterns and staffing, and rewards and incentives—indicate clearly that developing effective research operations in Japan will be a demanding task for a US firm. Each presents a significant challenge both to a US firm's organizational structures for its subunit and to its general technology strategy *vis-a-vis* Japan.

The Strategic Implications for US Firms

The linkage with manufacturing is perhaps the most wide-reaching in its implications. The close linkages between design and manufacturing explain why Japanese firms in this industry are perceived by engineering managers on both sides of the Pacific as more successful than US firms at moving products quickly from the design stage through development and manufacturing to the market with high quality and reliability. Indeed, the desire to tap into this kind of engineering expertise is often an important motivation behind the US firm's establishment of R&D facilities in Japan. But our study suggests strongly that this close linkage is not inherent in the formal training of Japanese engineers or in Japanese "engineering culture," but is due to the multiple linkages between design and manufacturing within the firm. If a US firm establishes stand-alone R&D facilities in Japan without a substantial manufacturing presence, it is unlikely to realize this key competitive advantage of Japanese R&D organization. Moreover, because the movement into line management in manufacturing is a standard part of the design engineer's career path in the Japanese context, the absence of a major manufacturing presence in Japan may well deter many Japanese engineers from joining the US firm, because of doubts about promotion and career possibilities.

The linkage between design and manufacturing is also an area of difference with significant implications for US firms in general, not just in terms of any operations they may have or plan to have in Japan. The quasi-market relationship that exists between corporate level R&D facilities and the operating divisions is one that US firms might do well to consider emulating. Neither unit (the R&D facility or the operating division) is completely bound to the other in terms of resource allocation, but neither are they mutually independent. The negotiation involved between the two in R&D budgeting and the enhanced status of the operating division as an "internal client" of the R&D lab increase the linkages between the two functions. The steady flow of people across the R&D subunits into the operating divisions is another element of the linkage that might have significant benefits for the technology interface within firms in general, not just within Japan.

The structure of the technical labor market and the difference in patterns of recruitment pose problems for the US firm (and indeed for smaller Japanese firms as well). A major foreign company can decide to emulate the methods used by the large Japanese firms: that is, to cultivate close ties with key professors at the top universities, so as to enter the allocation system. IBM-Japan has done this with great success, but it is a process that takes time. US firms may therefore be tempted to rely instead on recruiting engineers from the lower-ranking universities.

Such a strategy may have costs, however: the prestige of a firm is closely associated with its attractiveness to graduates of the top universities, and a firm that is seen as recruiting only from second-rate universities may itself be seen as second-rate. The prestige factor is sometimes one that is unappreciated by US firms, the more so because it is by no means clear that the education offered at the most prestigious universities is of higher quality than that at lower-ranking schools.

On the other hand, there are more immediate opportunities for recruiting mid-career engineers out of the major Japanese firms. Not all Japanese engineers wholeheartedly approve of the standardization of career paths. Some would prefer to remain in research roles in the central lab, rather than transferring to the divisions, but their only alternative to the transfer is to leave the company. This provides a "window of opportunity" for US firms attempting to set up or expand research facilities in Japan: Engineers from the central labs of major Japanese companies who are at the stage of their careers when they are facing a transfer to the divisions may be targets for recruitment into a research facility which will allow them to continue active research. There is also considerable dissatisfaction with the complete absence of immediate rewards for outstanding performance. In our questionnaire survey, Japanese engineers were significantly more likely than their American counterparts to express dissatisfaction with the level of financial rewards they received. This too widens the "window of opportunity" for US research facilities in Japan.

This should not, however, be taken to mean that US firms can simply apply their own patterns and expectations to the personnel administration of a Japanese facility. One implication of the general contrast in the locus of responsibility for careers in the two countries is that Japanese engineers expect greater career planning and company responsibility for their careers than their US counterparts. Even the "mavericks" who find the tight control of the large Japanese firm claustrophobic, and who are the most likely prospects for recruitment to a US firm will expect the company to assume more responsibility for their careers than would US engineers. This means that developing appropriate personnel strategies and structures will be a difficult and time-consuming process for firms starting up wholly owned research facilities. To completely adopt Japanese patterns of recruitment, career structure, and personnel administration would mean sacrificing one of the key competitive advantages of the firms in recruiting mid-career engineers. However, to transplant completely US patterns would likely produce great dissatisfaction and uncertainty among the Japanese staff. It is necessary to develop "hybrid" patterns, and this will take time and commitment. But the development of a coherent and long-term personnel strategy is a key ingredient for success in establishing effective research subsidiaries in Japan.

A Source of Danger

The differences in career patterns and incentive structures can provide yet another source of danger for US firms setting up research facilities in Japan. They may well look for research managers who have the qualities that make for successful project leaders in the United States. As a result, they may hire researchers who are technically brilliant, but who lack the skills that are essential for successful project management in working with Japanese researchers. They may also encounter problems when it is necessary to develop a cooperative working arrangement between a project group working in the United States and one working in the Japanese facility. The US researchers may quickly develop a contempt for someone who is a very effective project leader in Japan, but who lacks the technical superiority they value; the Japanese engineers may find it hard to work with an American project leader who commands the respect of his own subordinates by his technical expertise, rather than his management skills. An awareness of the different criteria of excellence in the two settings may go far in anticipating and dealing with such problems.

Finally, there is a set of strategy management issues confronting both the parent firm and the Japan-based R&D subsidiary. In the first section, we outlined the four major motivations behind the establishment of R&D facilities in Japan by US high-technology firms. They were: technology scanning to identify scientific and technical research that would be a significant input into the research process of the firm as a whole; technology scanning to analyze the technology strategy of Japanese competitors; research to tailor products to the demands of the Japanese market; and research that taps into the comparative advantages of Japanese science and technology to contribute to world-wide product development and the firm's overall technology strategy.

Each of these mandates has a different constituency within the firm. Central R&D headquarters is the primary internal client for the first, and they are likely to want technology scanning for research purposes to have a high priority in the activities of the Japanese operation. Competitor scanning is likely to have a different, but equally urgent client: those groups at corporate headquarters who are developing global strategy. The client for research that tailors products to the local market (the classic role of overseas R&D facilities) will be the local marketing organization, one whose demands may have especial force for the research facility because of its physical proximity. Finally, in terms of corporate budgeting and long-term survival of the R&D operation, making a major contribution in research terms to the development of new products for world-wide markets is likely to be the most visible and therefore highest priority activity of researchers within the Japanese facility.

Given the growing Japanese capacity in science and technology, and the nature of the technical job market in Japan, it is the fourth mandate—developing products on a world-wide basis—that would seem to be both the most effective use of the resources necessary to build an effective operation in Japan and the one which would be most attractive to potential Japanese recruits. But it is also the mandate with the least specific internal corporate constituency. Without a strong high-level recognition of the forces that make such a strategic mandate desirable, and a long-term commitment at the top levels of the US firm, it is unlikely that the time and resources necessary to meet organizational challenges of developing effective management and liaison systems will be available.

There is an obvious danger of overloading the Japanese research operation, especially in its early stages, when it is also struggling with the organizational problems of recruitment and of developing structures that combine features of US and Japanese research organizations. The choices made in these early stages are crucial for the long-term viability of the operation. For example, if the technology scanning activities take precedence, it will become increasingly difficult for the facility to attract first-class researchers. After all, the key pool of potential recruits to a new operation consists of the mid-career engineers from the large firms who are willing to leave the security of their current jobs for the opportunity to do challenging research instead of moving into line management. They are unlikely to be attracted by the prospect of technology scanning. Such recruits are, in turn, essential in beginning to build linkages with the major universities from which they were graduated.

In the long term, without people who are seen by the Japanese research establishment as "first-rate"—by virtue of their university background and their research activities—the Japanese facility will be unlikely to be capable of doing an effective job even of technology scanning: Its people will lack the access to the informal information networks of the research establishment that are so critical to obtaining and assessing timely information.

The first section of this article presented the factors that were pushing US firms into establishing or considering establishing research facilities in Japan. This section has laid out—on the basis of comparative research into the organization of R&D in the Japanese and US computer industries—some of the major difficulties that they are likely to encounter in doing so.

Clearly, this list of potential problems indicates that building effective research facilities in Japan will be a slow and difficult process for US firms, and will involve major commitments from them.

The importance of Japan as a market, as the home base of major internationally competitive firms, and as a source of new technology, however, requires that US technology-intensive corporations take the time and effort to seriously consider development of such facilities and the organizational systems to support them, if these firms wish to remain genuinely "global players" in technology.

Notes

1. Robert Ronstadt and Robert J. Kramer, "Internationalizing Industrial Innovation," *Journal of Business Strategy*, Vol. 3, no. 3 (Winter 1983), pp. 3–15.
2. See "A Global Reach in the R&D Realm," *Datamation* 30 (April 1, 1984), pp. 153–156.
3. See for example the observation of Jules J. Duga, principal research scientist at Battelle Memorial Institute: "The Japanese have obviously been much, much better than us when it comes to taking new technology and doing something with it." (*Business Week*, July 8, 1985, p. 87). This viewpoint was repeatedly enunciated by informants on both sides of the Pacific in the computer industry study cited below.
4. Robert Gibson, "Japanese Scientific and Technical Information", pp. 14–26 in *Japanese scientific and technical information in the United States (Proceedings of a Workshop at MIT)*, published by the National Technical Information Service, Department of Commerce, (PB83-179903); also Kagaku gijutsu-cho (Science and Technology Agency), *Kagaku gijutsu hakusho (Showa 58)* (Science and Technology White Paper, 1983) published in Tokyo by the Okura-sho.
5. This is not a new development. A British engineer, Henry Dyer, writing in 1904, noted that "Japanese engineers and scientific men are often found better informed regarding the contents of British journals than are many in this country." From *Dai Nippon: A Study in National Evolution* (London: Blackie and Son, Ltd., 1904), p. 176.
6. Leonard Lynn, "Technology Transfer to Japan: What We Know, What We Need to Know, and What We Know That May Not Be So," paper given at the SSRC Conference on International Technology Transfer: Concepts, Measures, and Comparisons, June 2–3, 1983, New York City. We should make it clear that while Lynn cites examples of this viewpoint, his paper is largely a critique of the lack of solid evidence for it.
7. See the transcript of the testimony at these hearings published under the title of "The Availability of Japanese Scientific and Technical Information in the United States," hearings before the Subcommittee on Science, Research, and Technology of the Committee on Science and Technology of the House of Representatives, March 6, 7, 1984 (Washington: US Government Printing Office, 1984).
8. See data from the Prime Minister's Office cited in Lynn, *op. cit.*, p. 8.
9. See the series of annual White Papers on Science and Technology (*Kagaku Gijutsu Hakusho*) published by the Science and Technology Agency, especially those for 1983 and 1984.
10. In 1981, the US government share of the nation's total R&D expenditures (non-defence-related) was 30.3%; in West Germany it is 40.9%; in France, 46.7%; and in Japan, 24.5%. OECD data, published in the Kagaku Gijutsu-cho, *Kagaku gijutsu yoran* (Indicators of Science and Technology), Tokyo, 1983.
11. *Business Week*, Feb. 25, 1985, p. 96.
12. See, for example, the Battelle Memorial Institute report for the US Department of Energy on ten energy-related areas of science and technology in Japan: G.J. Hane, P.M. Lewis, R.A. Hutchinson, B. Rubinger, and A. Willis, "Assessment of Technical Strengths and Information Flow of Energy Conservation Research in Japan", Vol. 1, (Richland, WA: Pacific Northwest Laboratory [PLN-5244 Vol. 1], September 1984).
13. Gibson, *op. cit.*, p. 17.
14. Congressional Hearings testimony, March 1984, cited above; pp. 324, 342.
15. The suggestion that immediate steps should be taken by the US government to begin to remedy this lack of cultivation of networks with Japan's scientific community is one of the recommendations of the Battelle Memorial Institute study cited above (Hane *et al.*, pp. 17–19).
16. See the survey of Japanese efforts in this area written by George B. Kenney and H. Kent Bowen, "High Tech Ceramics in Japan: Current and Future Markets", *American Ceramics Society Bulletin*, Vol. 62, no. 5 (May 1983), pp. 590–596.
17. Among the major empirical research studies have been: Ronald Dore, *British Factory Japanese Factory* (Berkeley: University of California Press, 1973); Rodney C. Clark, *The Japanese Company* (New Haven: Yale University Press, 1979); Robert E. Cole, *Work, Mobility, and Participation* (Berkeley: University of California Press,

1980); Satoshi Kamata, *Japan in the Passing Lane: An Insider's Account of Life in a Japanese Auto Factory* (New York: Pantheon Books, 1982).

18. The study involved interviews in each company with research managers, personnel managers, and individual engineers. More aggregate data were collected through questionnaires administered to a stratified sample of engineers working in development projects in the companies. There were a total of 206 questionnaire respondents in the Japanese central research labs and 98 in the divisional labs; and 103 US respondents. The data presented in this paper use the responses from the central R&D labs, because the emphasis in US firms setting up research facilities in Japan, which are more analogous to the central labs than to the divisional labs. The research was carried out under the auspices of the MIT-Japan Science and Technology Program and the Harvard Program on US-Japan Relations, and funded by a research grant from the Digital Equipment Corporation.